OSCE in Pediatrics

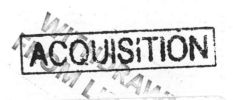

OSCE in Pediatrics

Second Edition

Vivek Jain
MBBS MRCPCH
Additional Director and Head
Department of Neonatology
Fortis Hospital
Shalimar Bagh, New Delhi, India

Manish Mittal
DCH DNB Fellowship in Neonatology
Consultant and In-Charge
Department of Neonatology
Cocoon Hospital
Jaipur, Rajasthan, India

RG Holla
MBBS MD DM
New Delhi, India

Foreword
Ajay Gambhir

JAYPEE   *The Health Sciences Publisher*

New Delhi | London | Philadelphia | Panama

Jaypee Brothers Medical Publishers (P) Ltd

Headquarters

Jaypee Brothers Medical Publishers (P) Ltd
4838/24, Ansari Road, Daryaganj
New Delhi 110 002, India
Phone: +91-11-43574357
Fax: +91-11-43574314
Email: jaypee@jaypeebrothers.com

Overseas Offices

J.P. Medical Ltd
83 Victoria Street, London
SW1H 0HW (UK)
Phone: +44-2031708910
Fax: +44 (0)20 3008 6180
Email: info@jpmedpub.com

Jaypee Medical Inc
325 Chestnut Street
Suite 412, Philadelphia, PA 19106, USA
Phone: +1 267-519-9789
Email: support@jpmedus.com

Jaypee-Highlights Medical Publishers Inc
City of Knowledge, Bld. 235, 2nd Floor, Clayton
Panama City, Panama
Phone: +1 507-301-0496
Fax: +1 507-301-0499
Email: cservice@jphmedical.com

Jaypee Brothers Medical Publishers (P) Ltd
17/1-B Babar Road, Block-B, Shaymali
Mohammadpur, Dhaka-1207
Bangladesh
Mobile: +08801912003485
Email: jaypeedhaka@gmail.com

Jaypee Brothers Medical Publishers (P) Ltd
Bhotahity, Kathmandu, Nepal
Phone: +977-9741283608
Email: kathmandu@jaypeebrothers.com

Website: www.jaypeebrothers.com
Website: www.jaypeedigital.com

OCSE in Pediatrics

First Edition: 2011

Second Edition: **2016**

ISBN 978-93-85891-67-0

Printed at Sanat Printers

Dedicated to

Our Parents
Mrs Sushila and Mr Suresh Chand Jain
Mrs Usha and Mr Mahesh Chand Mittal
and
Mrs Shantha and Mr BV Holla

Foreword

The objective structured clinical examination (OSCE) is an integral part of final exit examination for the postgraduate students. It is currently used by Diplomate of National Board (DNB) in a few specialties of medicine and surgery to assess the overall knowledge and practical skills of a student who is going to pursue his/her career in that particular field. It is also an integral part of examination for award of Member of Royal College of Paediatrics and Child Health (MRCPCH).

The OSCE system is in addition to traditional method of examining students (long and short clinical cases). This system has an added advantage of analyzing a student's knowledge over larger area in limited timespan. Also, to eliminate bias, all the students are examined on same set of questions simultaneously.

It has been commonly seen that the students are very apprehensive while undertaking OSCE examination, partly due to lack of practise and partly because of experiences shared by their seniors who have undergone the OSCE test. Nowadays, many institutes, where DNB courses are going on, have started focussing over this aspect and have started conducting mock OSCE drills for their students, which is quite encouraging and rewarding for the candidates undertaking their final examination. The second edition of *OSCE in Pediatrics* will be very helpful for them, especially after seeing tremendous response for the first edition.

Dr Jain is a Member of Royal College of Paediatrics and Child Health, London, UK, and Dr Mittal has been awarded Diplomate of National Board in Pediatrics. Both of them have personally undertaken OSCE examination for award of their degrees.

The book will be of great help for DNB candidates, other postgraduate students and also for practicing pediatricians.

Ajay Gambhir MD
President
National Neonatology Forum

Preface to the Second Edition

In response to the success of the first edition of *OSCE in Pediatrics*, we have come up with this updated second edition. On the basis of feedback, changes are made in the text matter of the first edition.

Medical science is ever evolving and new information is added every day. We have added more than 150 new questions to keep abreast of the recent advances.

The objective remains the same from the first edition. We regret any inadvertent shortcoming, and welcome suggestions and criticisms.

Vivek Jain
Manish Mittal
RG Holla

Preface to the First Edition

The traditional case presentation, still in vogue in most postgraduate examinations, covers only a part of the examinee's medical knowledge. The direction that the discussion takes during a case presentation and the level of interrogation depends both upon the examinee's and examiner's approach. This leads to a subjective assessment. Certain areas of clinical pediatrics, such as interpretation of laboratory and radiological reports, communication skills, problem solving, and knowledge of clinical procedures, are not tested routinely in the traditional examination.

The objective structured clinical examination (OSCE) attempts to overcome these drawbacks by providing a broad-based format to assess the candidate on multiple aspects of the subject. Objectivity brings with it an element of uniformity. Being structured gives a focus on preparation and assessment. The wide variety of topics inherent to childhood illness (from neonatology to adolescent medicine, from intensive care to social pediatrics, from child development to surgical emergencies and so on...) provides a delightfully wide source for the examiner to draw upon, but is a nightmare for the candidate. However, there is a silver lining. Being broad based, OSCE gives the candidate an opportunity to make up from an easy question, any marks lost in a station in which he has not scored well.

With the introduction of the OSCE system as an integral part of the DNB Pediatrics Examination, there was a felt need amongst students for a guide which could help them prepare for the examination. Moreover, the requirement to qualify separately in OSCE in order to receive accreditation made the necessity for such a volume all the more imperative.

The book *OSCE in Pediatrics* is neither meant to cover the whole field of pediatrics nor is it intended to serve as a question bank. It is an effort to sensitize and introduce the student to the OSCE format so that the student can prepare accordingly.

The ambit of OSCE extends beyond the examination hall. Preparation for OSCE trains the student to approach a problem in a systematic manner and would certainly help in dealing with the real-life patient.

We have drawn upon a wide variety of inputs in the preparation of the questions. No effort has been spared in trying to ensure accuracy of medical facts, drug dosages and so on. It is, however, possible in the changing world of medicine for error to creep in. We regret any such inadvertent shortcoming, and welcome suggestions and criticisms.

RG Holla
Vivek Jain
Manish Mittal

Acknowledgments

We must acknowledge the contribution of the following distinguished doctors, for providing inputs in the second edition of the book:

- Dr Akhilesh Singh, Consultant Neonatologist, Fortis Hospital, Shalimar Bagh, New Delhi, India.
- Dr BS Yadav, Consultant Pediatrician and Neonatologist, Cloud Nine Hospital, Gurgaon, Haryana, India.
- Dr Hemant Madan, Associate Director, Department of Cardiology, Fortis Hospital, Shalimar Bagh, New Delhi.
- Dr JK Mittal, Consultant Neonatologist, Neoclinic, Jaipur, Rajasthan, India.
- Dr Manas Kalra, Consultant Pediatric Hemato-oncologist, Apollo Hospital, New Delhi.
- Dr Manish Balde, Consultant Pediatrician and Neonatologist, Cloud Nine Hospital, Gurgaon.
- Dr Pankaj Kumar, Senior Consultant, Department of Radiology, Fortis Hospital, Shalimar Bagh, New Delhi.
- Dr Pritum Gupta, Senior Registrar, Department of Pediatrics, Cocoon Hospital, Jaipur.
- Dr Sandeep Dubey, Consultant Pediatrician and Neonatologist, Cloud Nine Hospital, Gurgaon.
- Dr Sanjay Wazir, Neonatologist, Cloud Nine Hospital, Gurgaon.
- Dr Sanket Goyal, Fellowship in Neonatology, Sir Ganga Ram Hospital, New Delhi.
- Dr Satyen Hemrajani, Consultant Neonatologist, Fortis Escorts Hospital, Jaipur.
- Dr Sourabh Singh, Consultant Neonatologist, Mahatama Gandhi Medical College and Hospital, Jaipur.
- Dr Surender Kumar, Consultant Pediatrician and Neonatologist, Cloud Nine Hospital, Gurgaon.

We also thank to Mr Himanshu Kumar for compilation and designing of data, graphs, etc.

Contents

Introduction

The objective structured clinical examination (OSCE) is an integral part of the accreditation examination for the Diplomate of National Board (DNB) in Pediatrics. It is conducted as a part of the practical examination, and is held on one of the three days of the practical examination (depending upon the number of candidates in a center). The OSCE part of the examination is held for all candidates on the same day.

The *OSCE in Pediatrics* conducted by the National Board consists of 25–30 stations that the candidate has to attend by rotation. Each station has one or more tasks for the candidate to complete in a fixed time, usually 5 minutes. The stations consist of questions or problems and usually cover the following topics:

1. Case studies.
2. Interpretation of laboratory reports.
3. Interpretation of radiological investigations, which may be conventional radiographs, ultrasonograms, CT scans or MRIs.
4. Interpretation of ECGs.
5. Clinical photographs.
6. Biostatistics problems.
7. Questions in community medicine related to pediatircs/neonatology.
8. Observed stations—at these stations, an examiner observes the actions of the candidate while performing a task. The task given may be one of the following:
   a. A situation in neonatal resuscitation.
   b. A situation in pediatric advanced life support.
   c. Clinical examination of a system.
   d. Anthropometry and derivation of indices of growth and nutrition.
   e. Procedure, e.g. liver biopsy on a dummy, etc.
   f. Counseling—includes counseling a patient to use a particular drug device or of a parent regarding a child's illness.
9. Drug or vaccine.
10. Equipment or instrument.
11. Biomedical waste management.

Each station is usually of five marks. The examiners are given a key which is their guideline for assessment. As such, there is no scope for an examiner to delve beyond the key to award or deduct additional marks for supplementary correct or incorrect information given by the candidate. Most answers are from standard textbooks in pediatrics.

Observed stations are a challenge but can be easily mastered with a little practice. Marks are awarded for each point covered by the candidate including introducing oneself and establishing rapport, taking permission prior to uncovering and examining a patient, covering a patient after having completed the examination and wishing the patient before leaving. In the history taking and counseling stations, the content rather than the style is assessed. The examiner expects basic competency and basic steps in history taking and clinical examination. Questions related to NALS and PALS stick to the standard guidelines. Thus, it is possible to score well in these stations if one goes prepared.

By and large, the laboratory and radiological investigations given in OSCE are simple and straightforward and stress on the clinical aspect of the illness. Diagnostic skill possessed by a trained pathologist or radiologist is not expected of a student.

Poor performance in OSCE is primarily responsible for a poor outcome in the DNB practical examination and results from lack of knowledge or preparation for the same. A candidate would benefit from regularly practicing mock OSCE drills. This does not have to always take the form of a formally organized mock OSCE. Informal bedside rounds, group study sessions, delivery room calls and so on, provide ample opportunity for students to pose a problem and assess each other and practice for the observed stations.

The final word for success in OSCE:
Practice, practice, practice.

Connective Tissue

QUESTIONS

Q1. A 10-year-old presents with chronic joint pains and poor wound healing. Birth history confirmed his mother had premature rupture of membranes. On examination he was noted to have a significant murmur, lax joints.

a. What is the most likely diagnosis?
b. What is the typical cardiac abnormality associated with above condition?
c. How do you confirm the diagnosis?
d. What is the typical scar found in this condition?

Q2. This 8-month-old male infant had deformities of the limbs since birth due to fractures of multiple bones.

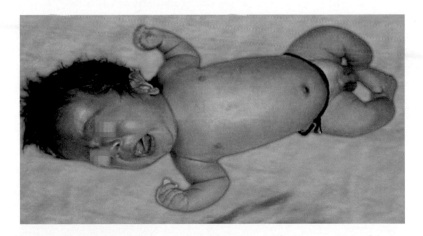

a. Identify the condition.
b. How is the condition inherited?
c. What is the biochemical defect?
d. What are the medical treatment options available for this condition?
e. What is the triad of this disease?

Q3. This 3-year-old male child presented with pain in abdomen for past 7 days (colicky), swelling over dorsum of hands and feet and pain in both ankles with swelling of right knee. Two days ago, the child developed a rash over the lower limbs.

a. What is your most probable diagnosis?
b. Which antimicrobial agent is used in the treatment of this condition?
c. What is the specific medical treatment for this condition?

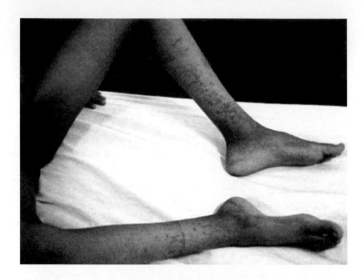

Q4. A 2 ½-year-old boy is brought with history of high grade, continuous fever, without chills and rigors, since one week. The parents deny history of diarrhea, coryza, vomiting or headache. Clinically, the child is conscious, irritable, febrile, normotensive, with no neck stiffness. There is conjunctival congestion, crusting of the skin around the lips and two discrete left sided cervical lymph nodes measuring 2 cm in size. Systemic examination is normal. The photograph of the child is shown.

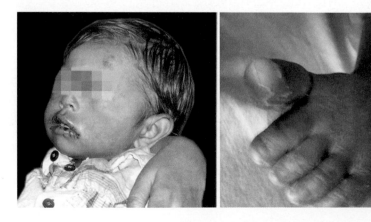

a.   What is your diagnosis?
b.   Name three laboratory abnormalities found on blood tests in this condition.
c.   What is the most common cause of death in above-mentioned patient?
d.   What drug (drug of choice) you would like to give to this patient?
e.   Meningitis can be one of complications (state true/false).

Q5. Male child aged 4 years is brought with history of painful swelling of both wrists, elbows, first metacarpophalangeal joints of both hands since 5 months, with low grade fever. There is no history of weight loss, rash, bleeding from any site or progressive pallor. Clinically, other than the swelling, stiffness and limitation of movement of the affected joints, there are no other significant findings.

a.   What is the most probable diagnosis?
b.   Name two investigations you would perform.
c.   Name three indications of the use of steroid in this disease.

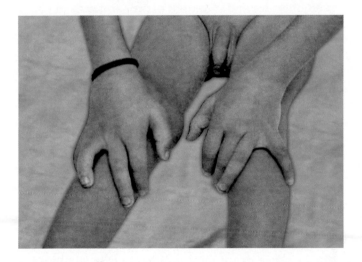

Q6. 2½-year-old boy was brought with history of sudden onset of limp followed by refusal to walk. The child was afebrile and there was no history of trauma. The child had been treated for an episode of loose stools with blood and mucus about two weeks back. Clinically, the child was afebrile, normotensive with no rash, lymphadenopathy, petechiae or pallor. The left hip was painful and movements were restricted. Other joints were normal. On investigations, other than a mildly elevated ESR, all investigations were within normal limits.

a.   What is the most probable diagnosis and what is the most likely responsible agent?
b.   Name the HLA positivity which is associated with this disease.
c.   What is the outlook for this disease?
d.   Name four viruses which are associated with arthritis.

Q7. A 14-year-old girl has been brought with history of high grade fever since three weeks with progressive breathlessness and swelling of feet and abdomen. The fever is not associated with chills or rigors, dysuria, coryza, jaundice or alteration in bowel habits. The child had a generalized seizure lasting for 2 minutes today. Clinically, the child is drowsy but arousable is pale, has oral ulcers, arthritis of both knees and a left sided pleural effusion. There is no jaundice or neck stiffness. The cardiac examination reveals distant heart sounds. The liver is palpable 4 cm below the costal margin and free fluid is present. A 2D echo confirms a pericardial effusion.

a. What is the most probable diagnosis?
b. What investigation would confirm the diagnosis?
c. What hematological parameters do you expect to find?
d. Name two drugs that can lead to this syndrome.

Q8. Five-year-old girl presented with history of insidious onset of weakness and fatigue on walking. Parents report that the child is particularly reluctant to climb stairs and is unable to lift her hands to comb her hair. The child has also developed a reddish rash around the eyes, over the dorsum of the hands and on the knees and elbows. There is history of joint pains of all the joints and the child has progressively restricted her physical activity. There is history of a upper respiratory illness a month back. Clinically, the child is afebrile, with no pallor, jaundice, petechiae. There is a papular non-erythematous rash over the face and limbs. There is generalized arthralgia, with no evidence of arthritis. Neurological examination shows proximal muscle weakness.

a. What is the most likely diagnosis in this patient?
b. How would you investigate to reach a diagnosis?
c. What is the treatment for isolated cutaneous lesions?
d. Bed rest should be given to the child (State true or false).

Q9. An infant presents with history of excessive irritability and fever since 1 week. He has been under treatment for conjunctivitis for the past 3 days with ciprofloxacin eye drops. The child is febrile (temperature 102°F, HR—150/min RR-38/min BP—100/60 mm Hg). He has a fine rash over his upper chest and his throat and oral mucosa is congested. His liver is 3 cm and is tender to palpate.

a. What is the most likely diagnosis?
b. What drugs would you use for therapy? Mention doses.
c. Name one finding on USG abdomen.
d. Name 4 common differentials for this condition.

Q10. A 26-days-old neonate is brought by the mother with a non-pruritic rash over the face and body noted since three weeks. The child has a heart rate of 60/min but is hemodynamically stable.

a. What disease would you look for in the mother?
b. What antibody is responsible for the disease?
c. Name two hematological findings one would expect in this infant.
d. What is the long-term outlook for the dermatological manifestations?

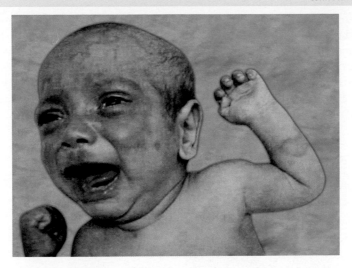

Q11.
a. What is the dose of methotrexate in juvenile rheumatoid arthritis?
b. Name two important side effects of methotrexate.
c. Which micronutrient supplementation is necessary while giving methotrexate on a long-term basis?
d. Name one skin condition where methotrexate is used.
e. What is the mode of action?

Q12. A 12-year-old female had a 2 year history of chronic sinusitis. She had one episode of hemoptysis and respiratory distress during the past 2 years. Urine analysis reveals hematuria.
a. What is the most likely diagnosis?
b. What laboratory test can help in diagnosing this patient?
c. What is the most important differential diagnosis for this patient?

Q13. Answer the following questions in relation to juvenile rheumatoid arthritis.
a. Name the monoclonal antibody to TNF alpha, used in refractory cases of juvenile rheumatoid arthritis.
b. What is the drug of choice for long-term treatment of juvenile rheumatoid arthritis?
c. What is the minimum number of joints involved to be classified as polyarticular arthritis?
d. MAS in context of JIA refers to minimal access surgery (State true/false).

Q14. This male child, aged 11 years was admitted with history of easy fatigability and jaundice and high colored urine of three months duration. Clinically, the child was ambulant, afebrile and normotensive. There was icterus, but no pallor, lymphadenopathy, cutaneous bleeding or signs of fulminant or chronic liver disease. The liver and spleen were palpable as shown in the figure. Finding on eye examination is shown in

the figure. Other systems were normal. The relevant lab results showed serum bilirubin of 2.5 mg/dL, direct positive, SGOT 243 U/L, SGPT 676 U/L, serum alkaline phosphatase 465 U/L. Other investigations including hematology, biochemistry, coagulation profile and serology for hepatitis were normal. The child was born of a consanguineous marriage and had an elder sibling who had jaundice, was unable to walk properly and was improving on medications.

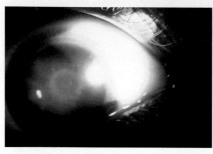 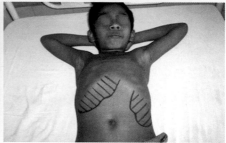

a. What is the most probable diagnosis?
b. What is the finding in the eye?
c. How will you proceed to confirm the diagnosis? Name three confirmatory tests.
d. How will you treat the child?
e. What dietary advice would you give for the child?

ANSWERS

A 1:

a. Ehler-Danlos syndrome
b. Mitral valve prolapse
c. Skin biopsy- collagen typing, lysyl hydroxylase or lysyl oxidase activity may be reduced. Collagen Gene mutation testing
d. "Cigarette paper scar".

A 2:

a. Osteogenesis imperfecta.
b. Autosomal dominant.
c. Structural/quantitative defect in type I collagen formation.
d.
   i. Growth hormone—improves bone histology.
  ii. Bisphosphonates (IV pamidronate or oral olpadronate)—decreases bone resorption by osteoclasts.
e. Fragile bones, blue sclera and early deafness.

A 3:

a. Henöch Schönlein purpura.
b. Dapsone.
c. Steroids.

A 4:

a. Kawasaki disease.
b. Thrombocytosis, raised ESR, elevated CRP, leucocytosis with neutrophilia, hypoalbuminemia.
c. Coronary artery aneurysm rupture.
d. Intravenous immunoglobulin, aspirin.
e. True.

A 5:

a. Juvenile inflammatory arthritis/juvenile rheumatoid arthritis (polyarticular type).
b. Rheumatoid factor, antinuclear factor, ESR, CRP.
c. During serious disease flare, bridging medication while changing to another line of treatment, intraarticular use for persistent limited joint disease, ocular control of uveitis.

A 6:

a. Reactive arthritis due to *Shigella*.
b. HLA B27.
c. Good.
d. Chikungunya, parvovirus B_{19}, hepatitis B, adenovirus, CMV, EBV, varicella, mumps, *Enteroviruses* (Echo, *Coxsackie*).

A 7:

a. SLE.
b. Anti ds-DNA, Anti-Smith antibody.
c. Hemolytic anemia with reticulocytosis, leucopenia <4000/cumm, lymphopenia <1500/cumm, thrombocytopenia <100000/cumm.
d. Phenytoin, sulfonamides, procainamide, hydralazine.

A 8:

a. Dermatomyositis.
b. Increased serum creatinine phosphokinase levels, SGOT and LDH levels and MRI of thigh (focal inflammatory myopathy) and muscle biopsy (perifascicular atrophy).
c. Hydroxy chloroquine (maximum up to 5 mg/kg/day) with low dose steroids (1 mg/kg/day).
d. False.

A 9:

a. Kawasaki disease.
b. IVIG 2 gm/kg slowly over 10–12 hours.
   Aspirin (initial 80–100 mg/kg/day q 6 hourly until 14th day of illness and then 3–5 mg/kg/day till 6–8 weeks after onset of illness).
c. Hydrops gallbladder.
d.
    i. Measles.
    ii. Scarlet fever.
    iii. Juvenile rheumatoid arthritis.
    iv. Drug reaction/toxic shock syndrome.

A 10:

a. SLE.
b. Anti Ro SSA, anti Ro SSB.
c. Neutropenia, thrombocytopenia.
d. 25% of lesions scar. Remaining resolve in 3–4 months.

A 11:

a. 5 to 15 mg/m^2/week.
b. Hepatotoxicity and megaloblastic anemia.
c. Folic acid.
d. Psoriasis.
d. Antimetabolite. Inhibits DNA and purine synthesis.

A 12:

a. Wagener granulomatosis.
b. ANCA and anti-PR3 (Proteinase 3—normally PR-3 is restricted to neutrophils granules but in this disease they are on neutrophil surface.
c. Churg-Strauss syndrome (Vasculitis—asthma, circulating eosinophilia and eosinophils on skin biopsy. There is no destructive upper airway disease).

A 13:

a. Infleximab.
b. Methotrexate.
c. 5 or more.
d. False: macrophage activation syndrome.

A 14:

a. Wilson disease.
b. Sunflower cataract.
c. Serum ceruloplasmin, serum copper, urinary copper excretion, hepatic copper content.
d. Restrict copper to less than 1 mg/day, D-penicillamine 20 mg/kg/day, zinc 25 mg three times a day.
e. Avoid copper containing foods: avoid storing or cooking in copper or brass vessels, liver, shellfish, nuts, chocolates.

Chapter
2

Counseling, History and Examination

QUESTIONS

Q1. A couple is sent to you by a gynecologist. Their first child is suffering from thalassemia major. Mother is pregnant again and wants to discuss options about the current pregnancy.

Q2. A 10-year-old thalassemic child is on regular blood transfusions since 6 months of age. He suffers from febrile reactions every time he gets transfusions. His pretransfusion Hb is usually from 6–7 g%. He is on irregular chelation with desferrioxamine using a pump. His latest ferritin level is 6000 ng/mL counsel him regarding transfusion and chelation.

Q3. A 10-year-old child has been diagnosed to be HBs Ag positive with raised liver enzymes (SGOT-73, SGPT-90) while he had presented with fever since 5 days. There is history of jaundice 2 and a half yrs back. How you will counsel regarding the reports to the parents?

Q4. A 42-day-old baby weighing 4.5 kg (birth weight-3.2 kg) presented with history of jaundice from day 6 of life. His total serum bilirubin is 11 mg/dL (Direct-8 mg/dL). Examination reveals firm liver 6 cm BCM, spleen 1.5 cm BCM, no ascites.

1. What important questions will you ask in history?

2. What investigations will you ask for?

Q5. A 5-year-old child presents to emergency department with red colored urine. Take the history from the mother.

Q6. Examine 1 day old term newborn.

Q7. You are resuscitating a newborn at birth. The baby has gasping respiration at 30 seconds after birth. Demonstrate what steps you would take for the next 30 seconds.

Q8. You have been called to see the parents of a child who has been recently diagnosed as a case of diabetes mellitus. Kindly counsel the parents about the disease.

Q9. A 10-year-old child presents to emergency department with hematemesis. Take the history from the mother.

Q10. A term baby is born by normal vaginal delivery; amniotic fluid was not stained with meconium. Go ahead with the process of resuscitation with provided dummy and equipment. You are free to ask vital signs of baby whenever appropriate.

Q11.
1. You are asked to counsel a mother regarding ORT (oral rehydration therapy) who's 9 month of infant has acute watery diarrhea.
2. Mother asks what to do if the baby vomits.

Q12. Take relevant history from this parent whose child is suspected to have urinary tract infection for the first time.

Q13. Perform hand washing.

Q14. Counsel the mother of a 7-year-old child who is being discharged from your hospital following acute severe asthma.

Q15. Obtain history from a mother who has brought her 5 years old child with history of unprovoked seizures.

Q16. A 5-year-old girl child is brought to ER with wheezing. She was diagnosed as an asthmatic few months earlier. What relevant history would you like to ask the mother?

Q17. The breastfeeding mother of a 3-month-old infant has come with request for advice. She has to report to work next week and will be away from home from 9.00 am to 4.00 pm. During her absence, the baby will be looked after by baby's grandmother. Counsel her regarding feeding the child and storage of breast milk.

Q18. You have been called in to counsel the parents of a newborn with meningomyelocele regarding the recurrence in the next pregnancy. How would you proceed?

Q19. You are attending to a high risk delivery of a HIV positive mother. The baby delivers and is hemodynamically stable. How will counsel regarding breastfeeding the baby.

Q20. You have recently diagnosed a 5-month-old infant to be suffering from beta thalassemia. He is the only offspring of his parents, who have both been diagnosed as carriers. Counsel the parents about the further management.

Q21. A 6-year-old child was brought with fever and hepatomegaly. There is history of jaundice 2 years back. Lab investigations have shown elevated SGOT and SGPT (56 and 88 U/L) and positive HBsAg. Counsel the mother regarding the investigations.

Q22. Examine and assess the patient with renal failure for volume overload or depletion.

Q23. A 12-year-old girl has been brought with history of recurrent headache since 6 months. Take a detailed history.

Q24. A female infant aged 14 months has been recently diagnosed as a case of simple febrile seizures. Counsel the mother on the disease and its management.

Q25. A 10-year-old girl has been diagnosed to have nephrotic syndrome. She has been started on steroids and has started showing response and is about to be discharged from hospital. Counsel the mother about the management at home.

Q26. Counsel the mother of a 4-year-old child who has recently been diagnosed as having acute lymphoblastic leukemia.

Q27. Teach an 11-year-old child with bronchial asthma to use a rotahaler device.

Q28. Teach a 9-year-old asthmatic girl to use a MDI device with a spacer.

Q29. A 6-year-old boy has been diagnosed to have celiac disease. Counsel his mother regarding the dietary management of the child.

Q30. A male infant aged 14 months has been evaluated for cyanotic breath holing spells and all investigations are normal. Counsel the mother in the management of the infant.

Q31. A one-month-old infant is brought to you with the report of a karyotype that shows that the infant has "non-dysjunctional Down's Syndrome". Preliminary investigations including echocardiography and thyroid profile are within normal limits. Counsel the mother.

Q32. A mother has brought her 19-month-old female baby weighing 10 kg with history of watery diarrhea since one day. The infant has some evidence of dehydration and you decide to give ORS (50 mL/kg over the next 4 hours). Counsel the mother.

Q33. A 2-year-old child presents to the emergency department with severe pallor. Take the history of the child from mother.

Q34. A 9-year-old child presents to emergency department with hematemesis. Take the history of the child from mother.

Q35. A 6-year-old child has been brought with seizures. There is past history of seizures. Take the history from the attendant.

Q36. Elicit soft neurological signs.

Q37. A 6-year-old girl child is brought to ER with wheezing. She was diagnosed outside as an asthmatic few months earlier. What relevant history would you like to ask the mother?

Q38. A male child aged 8 years has complaints of pain abdomen. Examine the abdomen.

Q39. A 2-year-old child is brought with history of coryza since two days and is now repeatedly pointing towards his right ear. Examine the right ear of the child.

ANSWERS

A 1:

Sl. No.	Action
1.	Introduce yourself
2.	Tell them that chances for a child being born with thalassemia major is 25% with every pregnancy
3.	Do genetic studies for parents
4.	Ask the mother the LMP
5.	CVS can be done till 13 weeks
6.	Risk of abortion 1%
7.	Amniocentesis can be done at 16–20 weeks
8.	Risk of abortion 1 in 500
9.	Parents may wish to terminate the pregnancy if found to be affected.

A 2:

Sl. No.	Action
1.	Introduce yourself.
2.	Tell the family that the transfusion and chelation practice being followed up by the family is grossly incorrect and will lead to severe sequelae of extramedullary hematopoiesis, chronic anemia and iron overload
3.	Keep pretransfusion Hb around 9–9.5 g%
4.	Use prestorage leucodepleted blood or use a WBC filter to avoid febrile reactions
5.	Use only packed RBC
6.	Ask them why Desferal was chosen for chelation and what are the reasons of intermittent infusion
7.	Tell them the optimal therapy will need 12–16 hours per day of infusion
8.	Give them the option of oral chelation with Deferasirox
9.	Counsel them that it has to be taken only once a day and chances that compliance will drastically improve with same.

A 3:

Sl. No.	Action
1.	Introduces himself and tries to make parents comfortable
2.	Explain the patient that HBs Ag positivity signifies that hepatitis B virus has infected the liver
3.	Hep B causes chronicity , cirrhosis and cancer (15–20 years later)
4.	It's a must to investigate this child-HBc IgM, HbeAg, HBe Ab, HBVDNA

5. Further treatment needed only if viral replication, i.e. HBe Ag–positive/HBVDNA positive
6. Screen family members with HBsAg
7. Vaccinate other family members if not already vaccinated
8. Fever not related to HBs Ag +ve. Repeat Liver enzymes later once fever subsides
9. No contact of his blood with anyone with a cut surface, no sharing of nail cutters/comb
10. Specify that there's no need for isolating this child.

A 4:

Sl. No.	Action

Ans. 1.
1. Any significant birth or antenatal history
2. Neonatal sepsis or hospitalization
3. Color of stool
4. Color of urine.

Ans. 2.
1. USG abdomen fasting to look for gallbladder size volume and then repeat after feed to look for contractility of gall bladder
2. HIDA after 5 days of phenobarbitone to look for excretion or non-excretion of dye
3. If HIDA excretory or liver biopsy is not suggestive of biliary atresia only then further investigation will be done to rule out underling cause of neonatal hepatitis
4. Liver biopsy to exclude biliary atresia, paucity of bile duct or neonatal hepatitis
5. Blood test: CBC, LFT, PT/PPTK, TSH
6. Urine: routine, for reducing substance.

A 5:

Sl. No.	Action

1. Introduces himself and tries to make the mother comfortable
2. Asks about duration of onset
3. History of blood in urine
4. History of associated symptoms: fever, pain abdomen, jaundice
5. History of swelling on feet or periorbital edema
6. History of associated pallor
7. History of bleeding from anywhere else
8. History of sore throat or skin infections in recent past
9. History of headache/irritability/seizures
10. History of oliguria
11. Diet history—beetroot ingestion
12. History of similar episodes in past.

A 6: Introduction to mother

Sl. No. Action

1. Cry/activity of child
2. Rooting/Sucking/feeding
3. Passed urine/stool
4. Look for any gross congenital anomaly (structural)/hernial sites
5. Temperature of child, specially peripheries
6. Look for icterus/cyanosis-color of baby
7. Auscultation of chest for respiratory and CVS system
8. Look for congenital dislocation of hip
9. Respiratory rate, breathing pattern
10. Umbilical sepsis/superficial skin infections.

A 7: Resuscitation

Sl. No. Action

1. Check Ambu Bag, mask, reservoir and O_2 source
2. Attach reservoir, and oxygen source
3. Correct technique of ambu bagging
4. Correct frequency of ambu bagging
5. Counting heart rate at end of 30 seconds.

A 8:

Sl. No. Action

1. Introduces himself and tries to make the parents comfortable
2. Explains: What is diabetes, type of diabetes and chronic nature
3. Management: Insulin, diet, lifestyle change, monitoring
4. Short term complications: Hypoglycemia, DKA, etc.
5. Long term complications: Renal, eye, cardiac, gangrene, neuro
6. Cause of Diabetes: Genetic/environmental/autoimmune
7. Risk in next child: Increased 3–6%.

A 9:

Sl. No. Action

1. Introduces himself and tries to make mother comfortable
2. Differentiate between hemoptysis and hematemesis
3. Duration of symptoms and whether its 1st time
4. What is the volume and color (coffee brown/red)
5. Bleeding from any other site/easy bruisability
6. Associated symptoms-fever/vomiting/jaundice/edema/abdominal distention

7. Associated seizure/mood change/sleep pattern change
8. History of drug intake NSAIDs
9. Any family history of bleeding
10. History of associated epigastric or retrosternal pain
11. Past history of jaundice/blood transfusion.

A 10:

Sl. No.	Action

1. Check supplies
2. Performs all basic steps in correct order within 20 seconds
3. Evaluates/ask for vitals
4. Decides for bag and mask ventilation (when examiner prompts hr<100/m)
5. Selects proper size mask
6. Position baby and himself correctly
7. Connects oxygen and reservoir
8. Appropriate ventilation (rate and rise)
9. Evaluate/asks for heart rate after 30 seconds and decides for chest compression (when examiner prompts h<60/m)
10. Locates compression area correctly
11. Uses right method of compression
12. Compresses consistently at appropriate rate
13. Check pulses
14. Evaluate/asks for heart rate after 30 seconds and decides for medication (when examiner prompts hr still <60/m)
15. Overall conduct of resucitation is fluent and is able to complete the entire process in given time.

A 11:

Sl. No.	Action

Ans. 1
i. Introduces himself.
ii. Explains that the main treatment is ORT and explains the need for rehydration.
iii. Explains correctly the preparation of ORT—whole packet in 1 liter of water.
iv. Advises feeding by spoon and discourages bottle feeding.

Ans. 2
i. Stop ORT for 5–10 minutes and restart feed, give slowly spoonful every 2–3 minutes.
ii. Advise giving small aliquots of 5–10 mL each time.
iii. Explains the danger signs of dehydration and explains when she should seek medical attention.

Does not become better in 3 days or develops danger signs (seizure/unconscious/rapid breathing, etc).
Encourage continuance of breast feeds/normal feeds/home available feeds.
  iv.   Checks, whether the mother has understood or not.
   v.   Ask the mother whether there are any doubts.

A 12:

Sl. No.	Action
1.	Introduces himself
2.	History of fever
3.	History of constipation
4.	History of urgency
5.	History of malodorous urine
6.	History of suprapubic pain
7.	History of loin pain
8.	Details of toilet training
9.	Wiping from back to front
10.	History of incontinence
11.	History of threadworm infection
12.	Family history of renal disease/stones
13.	Family history of UTI/VUR
14.	Note of thanks.

A 13:

Sl. No. Action

- Remove ornaments, watch, etc.
- Fold sleeves above the elbows
- Perform six steps of hand washing
- Palm to palm
  - Right palm over left dorsum
  - Left palm over right dorsum
- Fingers interlace palm to palm
- Back of fingers to opposing palms
  - Rotational rubbing of right thumb
  - Rotational rubbing of left thumb
    - Rotational rubbing of left palm
    - Rotational rubbing of right palm
- Perform in 2 minutes
- Air dry or dry with sterile towel or paper
- Discard towel or paper in black bin.

A 14:

Sl. No.	Action

1. Introduces himself
2. Clearly explain about asthma as hyperactive airway disease
3. Explain that there is no curative treatment and treatment reduces the severity and complications
4. Explain how to use MDI
5. Explain preventive strategies at home
6. Explain danger signs or warning signs of acute attack
7. Explain the treatment at home and to reach nearest hospital in case of acute attack
8. Explain the difference between rescue and prophylactic inhalers
9. Explain other alternatives, and ask for any doubts and clears it
10. Explain the need for regular follow up
11. Note of thanks and availability.

A 15: Introduces and establishes rapport.

Sl. No.	Action

1. Questions asked
2. Asks her to act out or re-create a seizure
3. History of aura and automatism
4. History of headache and vomiting
5. History of failure to thrive
6. Details of medications used that may precipitate seizure
7. Details of anticonvulsant therapy
8. Compliance of anticonvulsant therapy
9. Family history
10. Developmental history
11. Birth and neonatal history
12. Time of occurrence of seizures
13. Frequency of seizures
14. Precipitating factor like from fever
15. History of personality change
16. History of school problem
17. History of intellectual deterioration.

A 16:

Sl. No.	Action

Present History
1. When did the present attack start?
2. Is the child is getting better or worse or no improvement?
3. Does the child have rapid breathing, difficulty in talking or feeding?

4. Any factors that triggered the present attack?
5. What medications has she been administered for the present attack, at what dose and frequency?
6. Is it associated with fever?

Past History

1. How long has she been a wheezer?
2. How frequent are these episodes?
3. How many days the episode last?
4. Are these episodes seasonal?
5. How often symptomatic at night?
6. How often absent from school?
7. If child is on long term medications—if she has been compliant?
8. If using MDI follows the right technique?
9. How often she has to use reliever MDI or get nebulised?
10. History of previous hospitalization and if she needed parenteral or oral steroids/IV medications?
11. History of Frequency of visits to ER
12. Any admission to ICU and if so if mother has been told about warning signs
13. History of exposure to passive smoking/pets and other triggers
14. Is wheeze exercise induced?
15. History regarding co-morbid conditions like sinusitis, GER and other allergies?

Family History

1. History of asthma or atopy in family.

A 17: Counselling regarding feeding the child and storage of breast milk.

Sl. No. Action

---

1. Establishes rapport. Introduces himself/herself. Asks for a chaperone if male candidate.
2. Enquires about urination, adequate weight gain. Reassures about adequacy of breastfeeds.
3. Asks if mother is familiar with the technique of milk expression—if not, explains technique verbally.
4. Counsels correctly regarding expression and storing of breast milk: 8 hours in room temperature, 24 hours in refrigerator (non-freezer compartment).
5. Advises that milk should not be heated but allowed to come to room temperature spontaneously.
6. Advises to feed the milk with a cup and spoon or paladai.
7. Advises mother to continue with breastfeeding when she is at home.
8. Asks if mother has any doubts and encourages her to ask questions.
9. Wishes mother and offers a telephone number where she can have any other queries answered.

A 18: Counselling the parents of a newborn with meningomyelocele regarding the recurrence in the next pregnancy.

Sl. No.	Action
1.	Establishes rapport. Introduces himself/herself. Asks for a chaperone if male candidate.
2.	States that based on history, examination and investigations, a diagnosis of meningomyelocele has been made.
3.	Explains about the possibility of recurrence in the next pregnancy.
4.	Explains that the recurrence can be prevented by use of folic acid.
5.	Advises that folic acid should be started one month preceding conception in the dose of 4 mg OD and continued thereafter.
6.	Asks if mother has any doubts and encourages her to ask questions.
7.	Wishes mother and offers a telephone number where she can have her queries answered.

A 19: Counselling regarding breastfeeding of baby born to HIV positive mother.

Sl. No.	Action
1.	Establishes rapport. Introduces himself/herself. Asks for a chaperone if male candidate.
2.	Explains the benefits of breastfeeding for the baby. Also mention that the virus can be transmitted from the mother to the baby by breast milk.
3.	Explains the risks of not giving breastfeeding.
4.	Stresses the need for hygiene and exclusive feeding in case mother decides on either.
5.	Asks if mother has any doubts and encourages her to ask questions.
6.	Wishes mother and offers a telephone number where she can have any other queries answered.

A 20: Counselling the parents about the further management of baby with thalassemia.

Sl. No.	Action
1.	Establishes rapport. Introduces himself/herself. Asks for a chaperone if male candidate.
2.	States that based on history, examination and investigations, a diagnosis of thalassemia has been made.
3.	Explains the need for blood transfusions and hepatitis vaccinations for the infant and need to maintain the Hb above 9 gm/dL.
4.	Explains that cure can be achieved by bone marrow transplantation from a sibling.
5.	Explains to them that prenatal testing is available in the next pregnancy.

6. Suggests the role for cord blood collection from the next child, which can be used for stem cell transplantation to this infant.
7. Asks if mother has any doubts and encourages her to ask questions.
8. Wishes mother and offers a telephone number where she can have any other queries answered.

A 21: Counselling the mother regarding hepatitis B positivity.

Sl. No. Action

1. Establishes rapport. Introduces himself/herself. Asks for a chaperone if male candidate.
2. Explains that HBsAg positivity means that the hepatitis B virus has infected the liver.
3. Explains that hepatitis B can cause chronic liver disease which may, at a later stage, lead to cirrhosis and cancer.
4. Stresses the need to investigate the child further with HBc IgM, HBeAg, anti HBe and HBVDNA.
5. States that further treatment will be given only if HBeAg or HBVDNA is positive.
6. States the need to screen family members for HBsAg and vaccinate those negative.
7. States that there should be no contact of his blood with a cut surface, nail cutters, combs.
8. Explains that there is no need to isolate the child, or his utensils, eating, play or toilet area, etc.
9. Asks if mother has any doubts and encourages her to ask questions.
10. Wishes mother and offers a telephone number where she can have any other queries answered.

A 22: Examination and assessment of the patient with renal failure for volume overload or depletion.

Sl. No. Action

1. Introduces himself, asks for a chaperone (if indicated) and asks for permission to examine.
2. Checks tongue and axilla for moistness.
3. Checks ankles and sacrum for edema.
4. Checks for elevated JVP—in the sitting, semi reclining and lying positions.
5. Checks pulse and blood pressure. Blood pressure to be checked in lying and standing positions to check for postural hypotension.
6. Covers the patient and thanks him.

Imp: Do not waste time trying to take a history or doing a thorough general examination.

A 23: History for recurrent headache.

Sl. No.	Action
1.	Establishes rapport. Introduces himself/herself. Asks for chaperone if male candidate.
2.	Asks about onset duration, location, severity and progression.
3.	Asks about timing and duration of each episode, any precipitating events or relieving events, any change in the character of the pain during the past six months.
4.	Asks about quality of pain, throbbing, increases during straining, change in characteristics of headache.
5.	Asks about associated neurological features like loss of consciousness, seizures, weakness of any part of the body, visual, hearing or other cranial nerve deficits.
6.	Asks about any discharge from ears, difficulty in reading, toothache, features of sinusitis.
7.	Asks about associated systemic symptoms like vomiting and its pattern, fever, weight loss.
8.	Asks about past history of similar events.
9.	Asks about family history of headache.
10.	Asks about any investigations that were done and about their results.

A 24: Counselling for febrile seizures.

Sl. No.	Action
1.	Establishes rapport. Greets the mother, introduces himself/herself. Asks for chaperone if male candidate.
2.	States that based on history and physical examination, the child has been diagnosed as having simple febrile seizures.
3.	Explains that this condition occurs in some children, who are otherwise normal, between the ages of 9 months to 5 years.
4.	States that the seizure has a tendency to recur in case of future fever in 30–50% of children after a first febrile seizure.
5.	Explains that a doctor should be consulted at the earliest in case of fever or recurrence of seizures. Explain that other than fever medications, the child may be given short term oral diazepam during the febrile illness to prevent the seizure.
6.	Explains that the seizure generally occurs during the height of fever and that future episodes of fever should be treated by using antipyretics and tepid sponging as and when they occur.
7.	Explains that in case of a seizure, the child should be kept in the sidelying position and neck slightly extended. Stresses that no object or food or drink should be put into the mouth at that time.

8. Reassures the mother that the condition has an excellent prognosis for long-term neurodevelopment.
9. Asks if mother has any doubts and encourages her to ask questions.
10. Wishes mother and offers a telephone number where she can have any further queries answered.

A 25: Counselling of a case of nephrotic syndrome on steroids.

Sl. No. Action

1. Establishes rapport. Introduces himself/herself. Asks for a chaperone if male candidate.
2. Explains that based on history, examination and investigations, the child has a kidney disease called nephrotic syndrome in which the child loses protein in the urine.
3. States that the treatment for the disease has been started and that in a few days, the swelling over the body will gradually decrease and disappear. Emphasizes the need to continue treatment as per instructions from the doctor and that medications should not be stopped or modified without the doctor's instructions.
4. Explains that the child's urinary protein needs to be checked every day and result recorded in a notebook, which needs to be shown to the doctor at each visit. Emphasizes on weight and blood pressure monitoring on weekly/biweekly basis from nearby hospital.
5. Explains method of testing urine for protein using dipstick.
6. Says that the child's treatment will continue for about six months and that regime would be changed depending upon the child's urine protein response.
7. Explains that the child can eat normal home food and attend school. Emphasizes that the child should not take added salt for his diet.
8. Explains that the child should be brought back immediately if she has abdominal pain, vomiting, fever, recurrence or increase in swelling.
9. Asks if mother has any doubts and encourages her to ask questions.
10. Wishes mother and offers a telephone number where she can have her queries answered.

A 26: Counselling for diagnosis of acute leukemia.

Sl. No. Action

1. Establishes rapport. Introduces himself/herself. Asks for a chaperone if male candidate.
2. Explains that based on the history, examination and investigations, the child has been diagnosed as having acute lymphoblastic leukemia. Explains that this condition is a form of cancer of the blood. It is not

transmitted from any of the parents and they should not be blamed or made guilty.

3. States that the condition is potentially curable with treatment and that the treatment will continue for about three years.

4. States that the treatment would include intravenous, oral and intrathecal medications and radiation therapy and that would cause side effects like loss of hair, nausea vomiting, diarrhea, bleeding and recurrent infections, which may require repeated hospitalizations.

5. Explains that the child must continue the treatment regularly and report to the hospital whenever instructed.

6. Explains that subsidized rail fare is available to children suffering from cancer and to their families.

7. Asks if mother has any doubts and encourages her to ask questions.

8. Wishes mother and offers a telephone number where she can have her queries answered.

A 27: Use of rotahaler device.

Sl. No. Action

1. Establishes rapport. Introduces himself/herself. Asks for a chaperone if male candidate.

2. Takes the rotahaler device and dismantles it. Shows the parts to the child and shows how to reassemble it.

3. Takes one rotacapsule and places it with the clear end downwards in the slot provided.

4. Shows the child how to rotate the upper part of the rotahaler so that the capsule breaks.

5. Asks the child to let out his breath and place the mouthpiece of the rotahaler in his mouth ensuring that the lips are closed around the mouthpiece.

6. Asks him to take a deep breath through the mouth and hold the breath for a count of five.

7. Asks the child to check that no dry powder remains in the lower chamber of the rotahaler. Dismantles the rotahaler and removes the upper and lower parts of the rotacapsule.

8. Tells the child that he must gargle his mouth and throat with plain water after having taken the dose.

9. Asks if child has any doubts and encourages him to ask questions.

10. Wishes the child and offers a telephone number where she can have her queries answered.

A 28: Use of MDI device with spacer.

Sl. No. Action

1. Establishes rapport. Introduces himself/herself. Asks for a chaperone if male candidate.
2. Dismantles the MDI device and shows how it functions by reassembling it and releasing a puff into the air.
3. Teaches the child how to assemble the spacer and fit the MDI device to the spacer.
4. Tells the child to release her breath and place the mouthpiece of the spacer in her mouth, taking care that lips form an effective seal.
5. Presses one puff of the MDI into the spacer and asks the child to breathe in slowly over a count of five and hold her breath till a count of five. Repeat with second puff if required.
6. Tells the child that she must gargle her mouth and throat with plain water after taking the MDI.
7. States that the child must continue taking the medications as prescribed by the doctor.
8. Asks if mother has any doubts and encourages her to ask questions.
9. Wishes mother and offers a telephone number where she can have her queries answered.

A 29: Dietary advice for celiac disease.

Sl. No. Action

1. Establishes rapport. Introduces himself/herself.
   Asks for a chaperone if male candidate.
2. Explains that based on history, clinical examination and investigation results, the child has celiac disease, a condition in which the child is unable to digest wheat and wheat products.
3. Explains that the treatment of this condition is to exclude wheat and wheat products completely from the diet, in addition to items made from oats and barley for the rest of his life.
4. Names a few wheat containing materials not to be taken like atta, maida, sooji, dalia and foods like chapattis, roti, bread, biscuits, upma, noodles, halwa, etc.
5. States that alternative foods in the form of rice, maize (makki), jowar, bajra and sago can be eaten without any restriction and stresses that their nutritional value is as good as wheat products.
6. Suggests to the mother that the best way to control the diet of a child in the family is if all the family members adhere to the same diet so that it does not place a psychological stress on the child.

7. Explains to the mother that the diet will have its full effect in about three months.
8. States that the child would have to undergo repeated testing after a period of three months.
9. Asks if mother has any doubts and encourages her to ask questions.
10. Wishes mother and offers a telephone number where she can have her queries answered.

A 30: Counselling the mother for cyanotic breath holding spell.

Sl. No. Action

1. Establishes rapport. Introduces himself/herself. Asks for a chaperone if male candidate.
2. Explains that based on the history and investigations, the child has breath holding spells.
3. Explains that breath holding spells are a benign behavioral disorder that occurs in toddlers are usually predictable and are usually precipitated by scolding or upsetting the child.
4. Reassures the mother that the spells are not life threatening and do not signify an underlying illness.
5. Advises the mother that if undue attention is paid to the spells, the spells will persist or increase. Advises the mother that the way to reduce the frequency of the spells is to pay as little attention to them as possible so as not to create reinforcement.
6. States that if the child becomes unconscious during a spell, she should place him in a safe location in a sidelying position so that he does not aspirate his secretions.
7. After the child becomes conscious, the mother and other family members should leave the child alone for some time and not pay undue attention by refusing to cuddle, play, or hold the child for a given period of time until recovery is complete.
8. Asks the mother if she has any doubts and encourages her to ask questions.
9. Wishes mother and offers a telephone number where she can have her queries answered.

A 31: Counselling the mother having a baby with non-dysjunctional Down's syndrome.

Sl. No. Action

1. Establishes rapport. Introduces himself/herself. Asks for a chaperone if male candidate.

2. Explains that based on the history and investigations, the child has been diagnosed as having Down's syndrome.
3. Explains the chromosomal basis of Down's syndrome.
4. Explains about the developmental outcome of the infant.
5. States that the infant will have to regularly monitored for development of leukemia, hypothyroidism and other medical conditions.
6. Explains that the disorder can recur in the next offspring and that the recurrence risk is 1%.
7. Advises the mother that antenatal genetic testing will permit diagnosis of the condition in the next offspring. Advises that this can be done at 10–12 weeks of gestation.
8. Asks the mother if she has any doubts and encourages her to ask questions.
9. Wishes mother and offers a telephone number where she can have her queries answered.

A 32: Counselling regarding ORS therapy.

Sl. No. Action

1. Establishes rapport. Introduces himself/herself. Asks for a chaperone if male candidate. Praise the mother for bringing the baby to hospital.
2. Explains that based on the history and examination, the child has lost fluid and salt from the body.
3. Explains that these need to be replaced by providing salt and sugar containing fluids like ORS to the baby. No tea juices etc. ORS is the best medicine for this baby.
4. Shows the mother how to take a packet of ORS and dissolve the entire contents in the required amount of water (if the packet is for one liter, the contents have to be put in a one liter bottle of water. If the packet is for 200 mL, the amount will be shown on a glass).
5. Asks the mother to repeat the procedure in front of him.
6. Tells the mother that the ORS can be stored for 8 hours at room temperature and for 24 hours in the refrigerator.
7. Tells the mother that the ORS is to be fed to the child in small sips with a katori spoon or paladai. Shows the approximate level up to which the mother has to give ORS in the next four hours (500 mL).
8. Tells the mother that there may be a transient increase in stools or vomiting when ORS is started. Tells the mother that she should continue giving ORS. Asks mother to monitor the stool, urine and vomit output.
9. Asks the mother if she has any doubts and encourages her to ask questions.
10. Wishes mother and offers a telephone number where she can have her queries answered.

A 33: History for severe pallor.

Sl. No.	Action
1.	Establishes rapport. Introduces himself/herself. Asks for a chaperone if male candidate.
2.	Asks about onset of pallor—sudden or gradual.
3.	Asks about history of any bleeding or bluish spots on the body.
4.	Asks about any history of associated symptoms—fever, weight loss.
5.	Takes history of jaundice.
6.	Asks for history of blood transfusions.
7.	Asks for history suggestive of worm infestation.
8.	Asks history of birth, community/geographical background, consanguinity.
9.	Asks about family and dietary history.
10.	Asks about history of drug intake.

A 34: History for hematemesis.

Sl. No.	Action
1.	Establishes rapport. Introduces himself/herself. Asks for a chaperone if male candidate.
2.	Explains about the difference between hematemesis and hemoptysis. Asks for color of blood-altered, fresh and volume.
3.	Asks about duration of symptoms and whether it is the first time.
4.	Asks about history of any bleeding from any other site including blood in stools or bluish spots on the body.
5.	Takes history of associated symptoms fever/vomiting/jaundice/ edema/abdominal distension/chronic cough.
6.	Asks for history of neurological problems, altered sleep pattern or mood.
7.	Asks for history of drug intake—NSAIDs, steroids.
8.	Asks for associated symptoms—epigastric or retrosternal pain.
9.	Asks about family history of bleeding.
10.	Asks about history of blood transfusion.

A 35: History for seizures.

Sl. No.	Action
1.	Establishes rapport. Introduces himself/herself. Asks for a chaperone if male candidate.
2.	Asks the attendant to recreate the seizure.
3.	Asks how the seizure started and what the child was doing at the onset of seizure to identify any precipitating factors. Asks for aura.
4.	Asks if the convulsion was focal or generalized, its progression and postictal stage, automatism. If loss of consciousness present then for how long.

5. Asks if the seizure was associated with uprolling of eyes, tongue bite, bladder, bowel incontinence, postictal neurological deficit.
6. Asks about associated symptoms—fever, failure to thrive, ear discharge, loose stools.
7. Asks about previous seizures, their type, frequency and treatment. Any investigations done in past especially neuroimaging and lumbar puncture.
8. Asks about history of anticonvulsant medications—dosage and compliance.
9. Takes developmental history- asks about any regression of milestones/personality or intellectual deterioration.
10. Takes neonatal and perinatal history. Enquire about family history of seizures.

A 36: Performs the following tests after introducing himself/herself and taking permission to examine from the patient:

Sl. No. Action

1. Tandem walking.
2. Disdiadochokinesis.
3. Synkinesis (mirror image movement).
4. Hand pats.
5. Repetitive and successive finger movement.
6. Arm pronation—supination movement.
7. Foot taps.
8. Hopping.
9. Elicit choreoathetosis by extension of arms.

A 37: History for recurrent wheezing.

Sl. No. Action

1. Establishes rapport. Introduces himself/herself. Asks for a chaperone if male candidate.
2. Asks when the present attack started and what is the progression of the attack.
3. Asks for history of rapid breathing and difficulty in talking or feeding.
4. Asks for any factors that triggered the present attack and about medications taken for the attack.
5. Asks for history of associated fever.
6. Asks about how long the patient has been wheezing and about frequency, seasonality, nocturnal symptoms and school absence.
7. Asks about long-term therapy, drug compliance and about correctness of use of MDI.
8. Asks about frequency of acute attacks, frequency of use of reliever medications/nebulization/hospitalization.

9. Asks about history of precipitating factors, presence of pets, passive smoking in the house.
10. Asks about associated allergies, sinusitis, gastroesophageal reflux.
11. Asks about family history of atopy, skin allergy.

A 38: Examination of abdomen.

Sl. No.	Action

1. Establishes rapport. Introduces himself/herself.
2. Takes permission, undresses the child. Keeps genitalia covered with a sheet.
3. Inspects from the foot/head end for movements/peristalsis. Observes umbilicus. Inspects genitalia by briefly uncovering them.
4. Gently palpates the abdomen quadrant by quadrant, keeping the flat of the palm and fingers in contact with the abdominal wall.
5. Palpates the abdomen for liver, spleen, any masses. Does bimanual palpation of the kidneys.
6. Palpates the genitalia and hernia sites.
7. Percusses the abdomen for presence of free fluid. Percusses for bladder dullness. Percusses the renal angles.
8. Auscultates four quadrants of the abdomen.
9. Covers the child and thanks him.

A 39: Examination of ear.

Sl. No.	Action

a. Introduces himself and establishes rapport with patient.
b. Takes permission to examine.
c. Asks mother to hold child with one hand and head with other.
d. Starts careful examination of pinna and surrounding scalp.
e. Examines external meatus.
f. Checks otoscope for adequacy of light.
g. Pulls pinna horizontal and backwards.
h. Introduces otoscope gently held like pen with ulnar palm touching head of child.
i. Examines the ear drum.

Drugs and Vaccines

QUESTIONS

Q1.

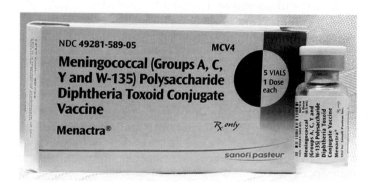

a. What is the usage of above drug?
b. What is the preferred route of administration?
c. What is the dose?
d. What is the minimum safe age?
e. What is the limitation?

Q2.

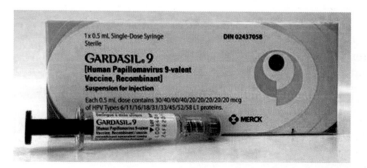

a. What is the usage of above drug?
b. What is the preferred route of administration?
c. What is the dose?
d. What is the minimum safe age?

Q3. A mother was worried that her newborn baby did not receive polio drops along with BCG before discharge from hospital.
a. What is the role of zero dose polio?
b. What is the content of oral polio vaccine per dose?
c. Unlike other live vaccines which are administered as single doses, why multiple dose of OPV are recommended?
d. What specific instruction has to be given to the mother after OPV administration?

Q4. DRUG: METHYLENE BLUE.
a. Name two conditions where it can be used.
b. Name two contraindications for its use.
c. What is the color of urine when a patient is given methylene blue?

Q5. DRUG: PARACETAMOL.
a. What are the indications for its usage? Name the different routes and dose to be given.
b. How frequently can you give this drug and what is the maximum dose limit?
c. What can be done to prevent toxicity?
d. What is the antidote for paracetamol toxicity? What dose of the antidote should be given?

Q6. Answer the following questions.
a. What vaccination schedule would you offer to a newborn baby born to a HbsAg +ve mother and when?
b. Which vaccine would you advise a thalassemic patient who is undergoing a splenectomy?
c. What is the minimum duration advised between vaccination and splenectomy?
d. Write the vaccination schedule for a person who has been bitten by a dog 3 hours back. The patient had been bitten by the same animal 1 year back and has received a full course of vaccinations at that time.

Q7. DRUG: ADRENALINE.
a. What is the strength (in terms of mg/mL) of the commercially available adrenaline ampoule?
b. What are the indications for its usage in NRP?
c. Name the route and dose to be given in NRP.
d. How frequently can it be given?
e. Give 3 noncardiac uses of this drug.
f. Give 3 cardiac and 3 noncardiac side effects of this drug.
g. Give 3 conditions where use of adrenaline is relatively contraindicated.

Q8. DRUG: AMPHOTERICIN B.

a. Mention one indication other than as an antifungal agent.
b. What is the maximum IV dose (mg/kg/day)?
c. Amphotericin B can be gives through oral route. Write true/false.
d. Most common side affect of amphotericin B therapy (name the system affected).
e. Which of the following is *not* the side effect of amphotericin B?
   i. Hypokalemia
   ii. Hyperkalemia
   iii. Hypomagnesemia
   iv. Hypermagnesemia.

Q9. RABIES VACCINE.

a. A pet vaccinated dog has bitten a child on his left leg. In this incident, the child got an abrasion of 1.5 cm with slight oozing of blood. What class of rabies exposure is this?
b. Which of the following is most essential in rabies postexposure prophylaxis?
   1. Local wound irrigation with soap and water.
   2. Antirabies vaccination.
   3. Rabies immunoglobulin administration.
   4. Observation of dog.
c. What is dose and route of equine rabies immunoglobulin administration?
d. A five-year-old child has received full postexposure prophylaxis for rabies 3 years back. Now this child has been bitten by stray dog and got class III bite. Which schedule will you use?

Q10. DRUG: INDOMETHACIN.

a. Write the dose and schedule of indomethacin given for the closure of PDA in a newborn who is less than 48 hours old.
b. Name another condition which can be prevented by administration of indomethacin in a preterm newborn.
c. Mention four main contraindications to the use of indomethacin.

Q11. DRUG: SODIUM NITROPRUSSIDE.

a. What is the indication for the use of sodium nitroprusside?
b. What is its mechanism of action?
c. What two specific precautions will you take while administering it?

Q12. Match the drug with the organism against which it is most effective.

a. Ceftazidime   1. *Mycoplasma*
b. Cotrimoxazole   2. *Pneumocystis carinii*
c. Crystalline penicillin   3. *Cl. difficile*
d. Vancomycin   4. *Pseudomonas*
e. Clarithromycin   5. *C. diphtheriae*

Q13. Answer the following questions with regard to storage of vaccines.

a. What is a cold chain?
b. What is a vaccine carrier?

c. How long can you keep vaccines in a vaccine carrier?
d. What are the other factors which damage vaccines?

Q14. DRUG: IVIG.

a. What is the dose for management of acute idiopathic thrombocytopenia with intracranial bleed?
b. What are the adverse effects? (Give at least 4)
c. Name 2 other alternative drugs in management of acute ITP with significant bleeds?

Q15. List two absolute and two relative contraindications to the use of DTP vaccine.

Q16. Answer the following questions.

a. What is lyophilization?
b. Name 3 lyophilized vaccines.

Q 17. CHICKENPOX VACCINE.

a. What is the dose and strain of the vaccine?
b. Above what age are 2 doses recommended and at what intervals?
c. For postexposure prophylaxis within what period after exposure, should the vaccine be administered?
d. How long can the vaccine be used after reconstitution?
e. What is the indication for giving varicella zoster immunoglobulin in newborn?
f. What is the route of administration for the vaccine and immunoglobulin?

Q18. MANTOUX SKIN TEST.

a. What is the composition of tuberculin used?
b. After what duration does it become reactive following TB infection?
c. Mention 4 host-related factors, which can depress the skin test in a child infected with *Mycobacterium tuberculosis.*
d. When can a tuberculin reaction of ≥ 5 mm be taken as positive? (Mention 2 conditions).

Q19. A baby born to a HBsAg positive mother receives HBIG and HBV soon after delivery and at 1 and 6 months.

a.
  i. When would you recommend postvaccination testing for HBsAg and anti-HBS?
  ii. How would you interpret the results?
      - anti-HBs positive, HBsAg negative.
      - anti-HBs and HBsAg negative.
      - anti-HBs negative, HBsAg positive.
b. What is the strength of the HBV vaccine used at different ages and for the immune suppressed?
c. What would be the vaccination schedule for a 2-year-old child who has received only two doses of HBV vaccine at 1½ and 2½ months of age?

d. A 15-months-old child due for MMR has missed HBV vaccine in infancy. What would be your advice?

Q20. A 1½-years-old child is admitted and treated for HAV infection. Child has not received any immunization so far as he comes from a tribal area.

a. What will be the immunizations you would advise for this child and at what schedule?
b. Is HAV vaccine required for this child?

Q21. STORAGE OF VACCINES.

Vaccines are stored in the refrigerator in your clinic. Mention the correct place of storage of the following:

  a. BCG
  b. OPV
  c. Measles
  d. DPT/DT/TT
  e. Varicella
  f. Hepatitis-B
  g. Hepatitis-A
  h. Typhoid
  i. Diluent
  j. Ice cubes
  k. Ice packs
  l. Dial thermometer
 m. Water bottles

Q22. UIP.

a. What are the objectives of UIP other than the immunization?
b. Name the vaccines used in UIP.
c. What are the immunization targets in the UIP?

Q23. A 5-year-old boy is brought to pediatric emergency room by his father after being struck by a car. Examination shows a lethargic but responsive child with a large frontal hematoma and bilateral hemotympanum. No other injuries are identified. A computed tomography (CT) scans of the head without contrast is ordered. The child becomes very agitated and frightened when taken to the CT scanner.

a. Which one of the following drugs would you prefer to sedate this child for CT scan of head?
   • Ketamine.
   • Midazolam.
   • Fentanyl.
   • Triclophos.
b. What is the dose of the drug used for this purpose?
c. What is the dose of midazolam if used intranasally in children <12 years old?

Q24. An 8-year-old child gets a road side injuries with abrasions on the left knee with dirt on that. Child has received full vaccination including DPT/OPV second booster at 5 years of age. Mother wants to know regarding needs to tetanus toxoid vaccination (TT) at present.

a. What will be the most appropriate advice?
    i. No need to give TT at present.
    ii. Give TT one dose.
    iii. Give TT along with tetanus immunoglobulin.
    iv. Give three doses of TT at 0,1 and 6 months.
b. What is the schedule of boosters for TT?
c. What is the content of toxoid in single dose of TT?

Q25. Answer the following questions.

a. Name five drugs/poison which can cause miosis in the child.
b. Which of the following is used as an antidote for acute INH toxicity?
    i. N-acetyl cysteine.
    ii. Pralidoxime.
    iii. Pyridoxine.
    iv. Physostigmine.
c. What is the antidote for heparin?

Q26. A 5-years-old boy diagnosed as a case of steroid-resistant nephrotic syndrome presents to your OPD for further workup and management. He has already developed some features of steroid toxicity. You want to start him on cyclosporine.

a. What is the dose of cyclosporine in this scenario?
b. What are the common adverse effects? (at least 4)
c. Name one drug that inhibits hepatic metabolism of cyclosporine leading to toxicity?

Q27. DRUG : CALCIUM GLUCONATE.

a. What is the strength of elemental calcium in the commonly available preparation?
b. Mention any 3 uses of this drug.
c. Mention 3 side effects of this drug.
d. What is the dose in treatment of hypocalcemic crisis?
e. Mention 3 important treatment options for hypercalcemia.

Q28. DRUG : VITAMIN K_1 oxide.

a. Give the pharmacological names of vitamin K_1, K_2, K_3.
b. Name vitamin K dependent coagulation factors.
c. Give 2 tests to diagnose deficiency of vitamin K.
d. Define early, classical and late hemorrhagic disease of newborn.

Q29. Match the following:

Type of antigen	Examples
• Live bacteria, attenuated	OPV, MMR, varicella
• Live virus, attenuated	HBsAg
• Inactivated bacteria	BCG, Ty 21a
• Inactivated virus	Acellular pertussis
• Toxoid	IPV, rabies, HAV
• Capsular polysaccharide	DT, TT, Td
• Viral subunit	Pertussis, whole cell killed typhoid
• Bacterial subunit	Typhoid Vi, Hib, meningococcal, pneumococcal

Q30. DRUG: KETAMINE.

a. What is the dose for anesthesia for short procedure?
b. What are the adverse effects? (At least 4) .
c. What type of anesthesia does it cause and which part of the brain does the drug act on?

Q31. Answer the following questions.

a. What is GAIN?
b. For AFP surveillance a rate of >1/100,000 population in children aged less than 15 years is the best indicator for good surveillance system (true/false).
c. Palivizumab (monoclonal antibody) is used to treat infection with which virus?

ANSWERS

A 1:

- Immunization to prevent invasive meningococcal disease caused by
- *N meningitidis* serogroups A, C, Y and W-135
- Intramuscular injections
- 0.5 ML
- 9 months (in case of outbreaks; usually given after 2 year age)
- Menactra vaccine does not prevent *N meningitidis* serogroup B disease.

A 2:

1. GARDASIL is a human papilloma virus (HPV) vaccine that helps protect against 4 types of HPV- type 6,11,16,18.
2. Intramuscular injection
3. 0.5 mL GARDASIL should be administered in 3 separate occasions over 6 months (0, 2, 6 months)
4. 9 years.

A 3:

a.
  - Uptake is said to be better in neonatal period as there is no gut flora to interfere.
  - Transplacental transfer of maternal antibodies against poliomyelitis does not interfere with the seroconversion.
  - As it is the first contact period between the baby and the health care provider, it enables logistic ease of administration.

b. Each dose of OPV contains:
   Type 1: 3 lacs TCID50
   Type 2: 1 lacs TCID50
   Type 3: 3 lacs TCID50   *(Park's Textbook of PSM)*

c. Multiple doses of OPV are needed for satisfactory seroconversion. The seroconversion with OPV is affected by poor antigenicity of the vaccine, thermal lability requiring stringent cold chain maintenance and interference by enteroviruses in the gut for proper uptake of the oral vaccine. Each time only one subtype of polio virus can cause antigenicity, hence more doses are required.

d. The mother need not be given any specific instructions after OPV, except that she has to report for subsequent immunizations regularly.

A 4:

a. Antidote for cyanide poisoning and for drug-induced methemoglobinemia.
b. Avoid in G6PD deficiency and in renal insufficiency.
c. Urine and feces turn blue-green.

A 5:

a. Analgesic and antipyretic. Oral/rectal; dose 10–15 mg/kg/dose.
   Intramuscular dose—5 mg/kg/dose.

b. 4–6 hourly; 1 g/dose or 60–90 mg/kg/day.
c. Toxicity is described with chronic usage in normal range. If chronic use is required, consider reducing dose to lower end of the range.
d. N-acetyl cysteine. 150 mg/kg IV over 15 minutes followed by 50 mg/kg IV over next 4 hours then 100 mg/kg IV over next 16 hours.

A 6:

a. HBIG and hepatitis B vaccine to be given within 24 hours of birth at different sites, followed by hepatitis B vaccination at 6 and 14 weeks or at birth, 6 weeks and 6 months. If HBIG is not available, HB vaccine may be given at 0, 1, and 2 months with an additional dose between 9–12 months.
b. Hib, pneumococcal, meningococcal, typhoid.
c. 2 weeks.
d. 2 doses of the vaccine are recommended on day 0 and 3 only. Antirabies antibody titers > 0.5 IU/mL are considered protective.

A 7:

a. 1 mg/mL (1:1000 preparation).
b. Heart rate below 60 despite 30 seconds of effective ventilation and chest compression.
c. IV (0.1–0.3 mL/kg/dose of 1:10,000 dilution) and intratracheal (0.3–1 mL/kg/dose of 1:10,000 solution).
d. 3 to 5 minutes.
e. Used in anaphylaxis, bronchial asthma, securing hemostasis and in some cases of hypoglycemia.
f. Cardiac—palpitations, arrhythmias, hypertension.
   Noncardiac—pallor, tremors, headache.
g. Hypertension, hyperthyroidism, patients of angina, during anesthesia with halothane and to patients on beta blockers.

A 8:

a. Leishmaniasis/*Echinococcus multilocularis*.
b. 1.2 mg/kg/day.
c. True.
d. Renal.
e. Hypermagnesemia.

A 9:

a. Class III.
b. Local wound irrigation with soap and water.
c. 40 IU/kg, 100% at wound site if possible.
d. Only 2 doses at day 0 and day 3.

A 10:

a. 200 microgram stat followed by 100 microgram followed by 100 microgram at 12 to 24 hours interval.
b. Intracranial hemorrhage.
c. Poor renal function, thrombocytopenia, NEC, sepsis.

A 11:

a. Hypertensive crisis.
b. Vasodilator.
c. Protect the IV tubing from light and discard if color changes from pale orange to dark brown or blue.

A 12:

a. Ceftazidime   *Pseudomonas*
b. Cotrimoxazole   *Pneumocystis carinii*
c. Crystalline penicillin *C. diphtheria*
d. Vancomycin   *Cl. difficile*
e. Clarithromycin   *Mycoplasma*

A 13:

a. It is a system of transporting, distributing and storing vaccines under refrigeration using any convenient methods, from the manufacturer right up to the point of use.
b. A vaccine carrier is a thick-walled, insulated box with a tight lid with removable ice packs, used for carrying small quantities of vaccines to the peripheral clinics and fields for use.
c. Vaccines can be kept safely in the desired temperature, generally for 1 working day in vaccine carriers.
d. Heat, sunlight and freezing are other factors which damage vaccines.

A 14:

a. 0.8–1 g/kg/day × 2 days.
b. Nausea, vomiting, headache, allergic reaction, renal failure, blood transmittable disease, anaphylaxis in IgA deficient individuals.
c. Prednisolone, methyl prednisolone, dexamethasone, anti-D, dapsone.

A 15:

a. Absolute—encephalopathy, anaphylaxis.
b. Relative.
   i. Temperature of >40.5°C or more within 48 hours.
   ii. Collapse or shock like state present within 48 hours.
   iii. Persistent or inconsolable cry lasting 3 hours or more within 48 hours.
   iv. Convulsions within 3 days, with or without fever.

A 16:

a. Live vaccines in powder form (freeze-dried) requiring reconstitution before usage.
b. Measles, BCG, MMR and oral typhoid vaccine.

A 17:

a. 0.5 mL; live attenuated vaccine from Oka strain.
b. After 13 years (at 4–8 weeks interval).
c. Within 72 hours (3–5 days).
d. 30 minutes (should be protected from light and heat).
e. If mother develops varicella 5 days before to 2 days after delivery.
f. Vaccine-subcutaneous ; VZIG-intramuscularly.

A 18:

a. 0.1 mL contains 1 TU of PPD stabilized with tween 80.
b. 3 weeks to 3 months (most often between 4–8 weeks).
c.   i. Malnutrition.
   ii. Immune suppression by measles, mumps, varicella, influenza.
  iii. Vaccination with live virus vaccine.
  iv. Immunosuppression by drugs.
d.   i. Disseminated TB/military TB.
  ii. Children with immunosuppressive conditions—HIV/organ transplantation or on corticosteroids > 15 mg/24 hours for > 1 month.
  iii. Malnutrition.

A 19:

a.
  i. 9–15 months of age.
  ii.
    1. If positive for anti-HBS—immune to HBV.
    2. If negative for HBsAg and anti-HBS—give a second complete HBV series of vaccination followed by retesting.
    3. If positive for HBsAg the parent should be counselled.
b. • 0–10 years   0.5 mL or 10 microgram
    • >10 years   1 mL or 20 microgram
    • Immunosuppressed   2 mL or 40 microgram
c. Give only one dose of HBV to complete the schedule.
d. To start HBV vaccination and administer the 1st dose simultaneously with MMR at a different site.

A 20:

a. As many vaccines as possible can be administered to this child simultaneously following the IAP schedule and administering optional vaccines as per the mother's request
b. No need for HAV vaccine.

A 21:

  a. Top shelf.
  b. Freezing compartment.
  c. Top shelf .
  d. Middle shelf.
  e. Middle shelf.
  f. Middle shelf.
  g. Middle shelf.
  h. Middle shelf.
  i. Lower shelf.
  j. Freezer.
  k. Freezer.
  l. Top shelf.
  m. Side door.

A 22:

a. Objectives:
    i. Self-sufficiency in vaccine production.
    ii. Establishment of a functional cold chain system.
    iii. Introduction of district level monitoring.
b. BCG, DTP, OPV and measles for infants and TT for pregnant women.
c. Target:
    • BCG, OPV, DPT and measles in age <1st year and TT in pregnant women.
    • 100% coverage for pregnant women and at least 85% for infants.

A 23:

a. Midazolam.
b. For sedation—IV loading dose of 0.05–0.2 mg/kg, then either same dose q 1–2 hour or continuous infusion of 1–2 microgram/kg/min.
c. 2.5 mg (0.5 mL) in each naris (total 5 mg) using 5 mg/mL injection.

A 24:

a. No need of TT at present.
b. Boosters may be given at 10 and 16 years and thereafter every 10 years.
c. 5LF.

A 25:

a.
    i. Opioids.
    ii. Phenothiazines.
    iii. Organophosphates.
    iv. Carbamates.
    v. Pralidoxime.
b. Pyridoxine.
c. Protamine.

A 26:

a. 3–6 mg/kg/day q 12 hourly.
b. Hypertension, hirsutism, tremors, nephrotoxicity, gingival hypertrophy, seizure, headache, acne, leg cramps, GI discomfort.
c. Erythromycin, ketoconazole, fluconazole, verapamil, metoclopramide.

A 27:

a. 10% calcium gluconate.
    1 mL of 10% calcium gluconate = 9 mg (0.45 mEq) of elemental calcium.
b.
    i. Hypocalcemia.
    ii. Hyperkalemia.
    iii. During exchange transfusion in neonates.
    iv. Antidote to calcium channel blocker drugs (e.g. verapamil), $MgSO_4$.
c.
    i. Subcutaneous extravasation may lead to tissue necrosis.
    ii. Rapid administration leads to bradycardia and cardiac arrest.

    iii. Administration through improperly placed UVC may lead to liver damage.

d. Crisis (when serum $Ca^{+2} < 5$ mg/dL): 1–2 mL/kg IV over 5 minutes followed by maintenance: 5–8 mL/kg/day continuous infusion or in divided doses.

e.
    i. Volume expansion with isotonic normal saline.
    ii. Furosemide—1 mg/kg q 6–8 hourly IV.
    iii. Glucorticoids: Hydrocortisone—10 mg/kg/day.
       Methyl prednisolone—2 mg/kg/day.

A 28:

a. K_1—Phytonadione.
   K_2—Menaquinone.
   K_3—Synthetic (fat soluble–menadione: water soluble—menadione sodium bisulfite).

b. Factor II, VII, IX, X, protein C, protein S.

c.
    i.   Increased PIVKA II levels.
    ii. Increased clotting time.
    iii. Increased PT and APTT.

d.
   • Early: within 24 hours of life or in utero.
   • Classical: up to first 7 days (usually day 2, day 3).
   • Late: after first week (2–16 weeks).

A 29:

Type of antigen	Examples
• Live bacteria, attenuated	BCG, Ty 21a
• Live virus, attenuated	OPV, MMR, varicella
• Inactivated bacteria	Pertussis, whole cell killed typhoid
• Inactivated virus	IP, Rabies, HAV
• Toxoid	DT, TT, Td.
• Capsular polysaccharide	Typhoid Vi, Hib, meningococcal Pneumococcal
• Viral subunit	HBsAg
• Bacterial subunit	Acellular pertussis

A 30:

a. 0.5–2 mg/kg.
b.
   • Hypertension.
   • Tachycardia.
   • Hypotension.
   • Bradycardia.
   • Increased cerebral blood flow and intracranial pressure.
   • Hallucination, delirium.

- Tonic clonic movements.
- Increased metabolic rate.
- Hypersalivation, nausea, vomiting.
- Respiratory depression, apnea increased airway resistance, cough.

c. Dissociative anesthesia and direct action on cortex and limbic system.

A 31:

a. Global alliance for improved nutrition.
b. True.
c. RSV infection in children less than 24 months with chronic lung disease.

Endocrinology

QUESTIONS

Q1. Match each action listed below with the appropriate enzyme

a.	Adenylcyclase	1.	Is activated by LH
b.	5 reductase	2.	Converts androstenedione to testosterone
c.	17 α hydroxylase	3.	Converts testosterone to dihydrotestosterone
d.	20 β hydroxylase	4.	Catalyzes the first step in the production of hormonal steroids from cholesterol
e.	21 dehydroxylase.	5.	Cause massive adrenal enlargement when congenitally deficient, is associated with poor survival of the affected infants, and can lead to the formation of female genitalia in genotypic ally male infants

Q2. Match the following

a.	Menorrhagia	a.	Bleeding between menstrual periods
b.	Metrorrhagia (hypermenorrhea)	b.	Excessive amount of blood or duration
c.	Menometrorrhagia	c.	Excessive amount of blood at irregular frequencies
d.	Hypermenorrhea	d.	Menstrual periods >35 day apart
e.	Oligomenorrhea	e.	Menstrual periods <21 day apart
f.	Polymenorrhea.	f.	Menorrhagia

Q3. Match the urine odor with IEM

a.	Sweaty feet	1.	PKU
b.	Cabbage	2.	Tyrosinemia
c.	Musty smell	3.	Isovaleric aciduria
d.	Syrup	4.	Maple syrup urine diseases.

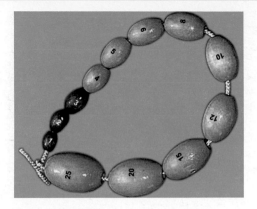

Q4:
a. What is the device called?
b. What is its use?
c. What is the significance of change in color?
d. What does number indicate?

Q5: An infant is being evaluated for DSD. You find clitoral hypertrophy and other signs of virilization. On investigations serum cortisol levels are low. ACTH and PRA are markedly elevated. ACTH stimulation test reveals markedly increased 17–OH progesterone. Serum testosterone is also elevated. Child also has severe hyponatremia.
a. What is your diagnosis?
b. What is the mode of inheritance?
c. What is the treatment for this baby?

Q6: A 9-year-old boy is brought because his mother feels he is short for his age. His height is 80 cm. His father's height is 160 cm and mother's height is 148 cm. His US/LS ratio is 1. 5: 1
a. What type of short stature does this child have?
b. What is the mid parental height of this child?
c. Name 3 causes for the short stature in this child?
d. What is the normal US/LS ratio at this age?
e. Name 3 conditions in which there is advanced US/LS ratio?

Q7: An infant is evaluated for seizure. The following are the lab reports.
Serum Calcium: 6.6 mg%
Po4: 9.3 mg%
SAP: 500 units
Mg: 3 mg%
a. What is the likely diagnosis?
b. What would be the levels of PTH and 1, 25(OH2) D3?
c. The same infant is also noted to be dark and having mucocutaneous candidiasis. What is the likely diagnosis?
d. CT brain is carried out. What finding do you expect in CT brain?

Q8. A 6-year-old girl was evaluated for excessive body weight. On examination she had weight of 35 kg and height of 110 cm. She had hyperpigmentation of axilla, groin and neck regions.

a. What is the body mass index of the child? If the BMI of the child comes at the 87th percentile, how would you classify her?
b. What does pigmentation denote? What investigation would you do for the same.
c. What musculoskeletal problems can this girl suffer?

Q9. A 15-year-old girl with normal breast development was brought with primary amenorrhea. External genitalia showed the presence of a firm labial swelling suggestive of a gonad. The vaginal examination revealed a blind ending vaginal pouch. On ultrasound scanning, uterus and ovaries were not detected.

a. What is the likely diagnosis?
b. What do you expect the karyotype to be?
c. What hormonal tests would you do and what results do you expect?
d. Should the gonadal mass be removed? If so why?

Q10. A 14-year-old female child complained of continuous abdominal pain since 10 days with bouts of diarrhea and vomiting for past 3 days. Since 24 hours, she has also developed weakness of both lower limbs and is unable to walk. Clinically, the child is restless, afebrile with pulse rate of 126/min, blood pressure 188/102 mmHg, diminished tone, power and reflexes in both lower limbs. Deep tendon jerks are not elicitable.

a. Give two possible differential diagnosis.
b. Investigations revealed Na—112 mEq/L, K 4.2 mEq/L, SGPT 37 IU/L. The patient is passing high colored urine—What is the probable diagnosis?
c. Suggest one investigation for diagnosis.
d. What is the treatment for this condition?

Q11. A 2½-year-old boy was brought with history of bowing of lower limbs and wrist widening. With the clinical diagnosis of rickets and investigations reports revealing total serum calcium of 7.6 mg/dL, serum phosphate of 3.1 mg/dL and alkaline phosphatase of 3000 IU/L, the child received a doses of vitamin D (6 lac units) along with calcium supplements. The dose of vitamin D was repeated after six weeks due to poor response in clinical, radiological and biochemical features. Further investigations show: 25 OH vitamin D 30 ng/ml (N-10-50), 1, 25 di (OH) vitamin D: 300 pg/mL (N-20-60).

a. What is the child suffering from?
b. What associated skin findings would you expect?
c. How would you treat this child?
d. What laboratory tests would you perform to monitor this child (Laboratory investigations).

Q12. An asymptomatic 11-year-old girl is brought by her mother with the concern that she is short and not growing. She estimates that the child has grown less than 2 cm in the past six months. There is no significant past medical illness or family history of disease. She is scholastically above average and is psychologically well adjusted to family and school. Her father's height is 170 cm and her mother is 160 cm tall. Physical examination reveals the child to be in B1, PH1, and no clinical abnormality is detected. Her height is 123 cm (< 5th percentile for age), and her weight is 28 kg (25th percentile).

a. Calculate the target height for the child.
b. What are the basic investigations you would like to order in this child to identify the cause of short stature?
c. Is there a role for growth hormone treatment in this child?
d. Had this been growth hormone deficiency, what clinical findings would you have looked for?

Q13. An otherwise asymptomatic 3 year male child is brought for evaluation of short stature. His height is 80 cm, the upper segment measures 50 cm and the head circumference is 51 cm. The proximal part of the upper and lower limbs are shortened in comparison to the distal parts. The face is mildly dysmorphic with mid facial hypoplasia.

a. What is the US/LS ratio. What is the expected US: LS ratio at this age?
b. What is the likely diagnosis?
c. What hand abnormality is seen in this condition?
d. What pelvic abnormality is seen on X-ray?

Q14. A 5-year-old girl weighing 13 kg has recently been diagnosed as having Type I diabetes. She has to be started on insulin at 0.7 U/kg/day.

a. Show calculations of regular and lente insulin therapy she should receive.
b. What counseling would you give regarding possible complication of insulin therapy?
c. This child was advised a diet having low glycemic index. What is glycemic index of a food?
d. What base line investigations would you do at start of treatment?

Q15. A patient being treated in the ICU has the following arterial blood gas report:

- Arterial blood gas
  pH   :   7.199
  PCO_2 :   38.4 mmHg
  HCO_3 :   12 mMol/L
  PO_2 :   86.6 mmHg
- Electrolytes
  Na   :   136 mEq/L
  K   :   4 mEq/L
  Cl   :   103 mEq/L

a. Describe the metabolic condition.
b. Calculate the expected CO_2 level for the given HCO_3 level.
c. Calculate anion gap.
d. Name two conditions with similar anion gap as above.

Q16. A 3-year-old girl presents with history of vaginal bleeding (2 episodes over the past 4 months). There are no features of trauma or local inflammation. On physical examination, breast development is at Tanner stage I. There is a café au lait spot measuring 8 cm × 3 cm over the abdomen. Similar spots are seen over the face, chest and abdomen.

a. What is the diagnosis?
b. What investigations will you do in this child?
c. What is the cause of the menstrual bleeding?
d. What are some other features you may see in this condition?

Q17. A 3-year-old boy presents with history of progressive penile enlargement and pubic hair growth over the last 6 months. The child is otherwise asymptomatic and of normal intelligence. Physical examination shows: pubic hair Tanner stage III, stretched penile length is 6.6 cm, testicular volume is 8 mL bilaterally. Other examination is normal.

a. What is your diagnosis?
b. What is the probable underlying cause?
c. What tests will you do to diagnose this condition?
d. What treatment will you offer?

Q18. A 4½-year-old girl is admitted with history of fever, vomiting and abdominal pain since 2 days. Clinically, the child is sleepy, dehydrated and tachypneic, with a heart rate of 122/min and blood pressure of 90/48 mmHg. Her blood sugar is 480 mg%.

a. What is the likely diagnosis?
b. The immediate treatment would be (tick the correct answer):
   i. IV normal saline.
  ii. 0.2% DNS.
 iii. 3 NS.
 iv. 1/3 NS with kesol.
c. What investigations from following list will guide you in immediate treatment? (you may select more than one answer).
   i. Blood gas.
  ii. Urine examination for ketones.
 iii. Sr insulin.
 iv. Sr electrolytes.
  v. C-peptide levels.
d. What CNS complication can you encounter during treatment?

Q19. Home monitoring of blood sugar in a diabetic child taking insulin prebreakfast and predinner, mixed split regimen (regular and NPH) reveals following:

	Pre breakfast	Before lunch	Pre dinner	Before sleeping 11 pm	3 am
Day 1	266	164	294	110	58
Day 2	284	168	278	118	72
Day 3	226	148	264	88	54

Contd..

Contd..

Day 4	258	204	274	146	76
Day 5	300	172	198	136	62
Day 6	248	182	212	140	78

a. What is the reason for morning hyperglycemia?

b. What changes would you make in insulin therapy?

c. When should the parents test for urine ketones?

Q20. Match the physical finding with the etiology:

Physical finding	Etiology
1. Disproportionate short stature	a. Growth hormone deficiency
2. Round head, small nose, small genitals, fine scalp hair	b. Achondroplasia
3. Round face, short 4th metacarpal, mental retardation	c. Cushing syndrome
4. Central obesity, striae, proximal weakness	d. Pseudohypoparathyroidism

Q21. A 13-year-old child came to the OPD with complaints of gradual loss of vision. On examination he had ataxia, intention tremors, loss of vibration and position sense. He had history of chronic diarrhea with passage of bulky frothy stools. His plasma cholesterol was 28 mg/dL and his serum triglycerides were 12 mg/dL.

a. What is the diagnosis?

b. What is the characteristic finding on peripheral smear of this patient?

c. What is the visual problem?

d. What is the mode of inheritance of this disease?

e. What is the most common differential diagnosis for this?

Q22. An infant comes to you for a 6-month well-baby visit. The mother says that the baby is very well behaved, hardly cries much and sleeps most of the time. She reports that during his first two weeks after birth, the baby had difficulty feeding and had many choking spells while nursing, which has now improved. Clinically, the baby has poor head control, no babbling, and is not yet reaching for objects. Physical examination shows a dull, sleepy infant with mild pallor and no teeth. The skin is dry and the muscles are hypotonic. The rest of the physical examination is normal.

a. What is your assessment?

b. What is the most common cause for this disease?

c. What is the risk if this condition is overtreated?

Q23. A 7-year-old boy is brought into the OPD because his father noted the presence of pubic hair. He is otherwise a healthy, active boy and family history and past medical history is unremarkable. On physical examination the child's height is at the 90th percentile and his weight is at the 70th percentile. He has moderate sebaceous activity on his forehead and nose and axillary hair. His pubic hair and phallus are Tanner stage III. His testes are 14 cc in volume. The examination is otherwise normal.

Review of his growth curve indicates that his height has increased from the 50th percentile at age five to its present level.

a. What is the most likely diagnosis?
b. What points from the history and physical examination are the most significant?
c. What diagnostic studies are indicated?

Q24. Answer the questions.

a. What is the cut off age limit for diagnosis of primary amenorrhea?
b. Which is the commonest CNS tumor responsible for primary amenorrhoea?
c. If FSH and LH levels are elevated, what is the etiology for primary amenorrhea?
d. At what SMR stage, majority of girls reach menarche?
e. A girl with primary amenorrhea presents with recurrent abdominal pain. What is the commonest cause?
f. Name one psychological disorder that can cause primary amenorrhea?

Q25. A 13-year-old girl is diagnosed to have graves disease.

a. What are the earliest signs in children with Graves disease?
b. What cardiovascular complications would you anticipate in this child?
c. Name 2 drugs used in the treatment of graves disease and mention three severe reactions they can cause.

Q26. An infant is being evaluated for a suspected inborn error of metabolism. The infant's reports are as follows:

Plasma NH_3—500 μmol/L ABG: pH—7.38 , PCO_2—42 mm Hg.

a. What is the most likely defect leading to inborn error of metabolism?
b. Give 4 examples of disorders in this group.
c. List 5 drugs used in treatment.
d. Which of these disorders affect males more severely?
e. Which is the most common form of these disorders?

Q 27. One-year-old male child 2nd in birth order brought to emergency department with chief complaints of vomiting and irritable behavior for the last 2 days and 3 episodes of focal seizures just before admission. Patient was given dextrose and calcium gluconate following which seizures subsided. Mother also says that her baby drinks liquids (including the breast milk) very frequently and passes urine very frequently. His weight is 4.5 kg and the a head circumference is 47 cm. His blood sugar is 78 mg% (sample taken prior to dextrose bolus) and he has pallor. His urine examination is positive for glucose (by dextrostix method) amino acids and phosphates. His blood gas is consistent with metabolic acidosis and

ionized Ca^{++} levels are 1.2 mg%. His serum phosphorus levels are low and Na is 135.5 mEq/L, K is 4.5 mEq/L, Cl is 105 mEq/L and HCO_3 is 25 mEq/L and alkaline phosphate levels are 886 IU/L.

a. What is the diagnosis?
b. What is the most probable etiology for this diagnosis?
c. What additional investigations you would ask for?
d. What is the treatment option available?

Q28. An 8-months-old male child is brought to the OPD with complaints of dry scaly skin around the oral cavity and on palms along with reddish tint of the hairs for the last 2 months. Lesions are increasing in severity since then. He was exclusively breast fed up to 6 months of life, now his is on top feeding (cows milk). His weight is 6 kg (Birth weight was 3.2 kg) and length is 68 cm. On examination he is found to have conjunctivitis, blepharitis, glossitis and stomatitis.

a. What is the most probable diagnosis?
b. What is the mode of inheritance?
c. What lab investigation will clinch the diagnosis?
d. What treatment will you advise to this child?

Q29. Fill the correct figures in the question given below.

Age	Upper: lower segment
Birth	
1 year	
3 years	
5 years	
10 years	

Q30. Match the table of bone age vs chronological age.

Findings	Diagnosis
1. Height age = bone age > chronological age	a. Growth hormone deficiency
2. Height age = bone age < chronological age	b. Familial short stature
3. Height age < bone age = chronological age	c. Simple virilizing congenital adrenal hyperplasia
4. Height age < bone age < chronological age	d. Constitutional delay in growth

Q31. A male neonate aged 17 days was brought to the hospital with complaints of excessive urination. Clinically, the neonate appeared dehydrated, with 22% weight loss since birth. Observation and investigations in hospital revealed the following.

Weight	:	2.8 kg
Urine output	:	479 mL/24 hours (>7 mL/kg/hour)
Serum Na	:	156 mEq/L
Serum K	:	4.2 mEq/L
BUN	:	14 mg/dL (5 mMol/L)
Serum glucose	:	108 mg/dL (6 mMol/L)
Urine osmolality	:	97 mOsm/L

Administration of a hormonal preparation failed to produce decrease in the urine output or change in urinary or serum osmolality.

a. What is the diagnosis?

b. Give the formula for calculation of serum osmolality. What is the serum osmolality in this case?

c. What is the treatment for this condition?

ANSWERS

A 1:

a. Is activated by LH
b. Converts androstenedione to testosterone
c. Converts testosterone to dihydrotestosterone
d. Catalyzes the first step in the production of hormonal steroids from cholesterol
e. Cause massive adrenal enlargement when congenitally deficient, is associated with poor survival of the affected infants, and can lead to the formation of female genitalia in genotypic ally male infants.

A 2:

A-1. Bleeding between menstrual periods
B-2. Excessive amount of blood or duration
C-3. Excessive amount of blood at irregular frequencies
D-4. Menstrual periods >35 day apart
E-5. Menstrual periods <21 day apart
F-6. Menorrhagia.

A 3:

A.-3. Isovaleric aciduria
B.-2. Tyrosinemia
C.-1. PKU
D.-4. Maple syrup urine diseases.

A 4:

a. Orchidometer
b. Measurement of testicular volume
c. Prepubertal
d. Volume in milliliter

A 5:

a. Congenital adrenal hyperplasia due to 21 hydroxylase deficiency
b. Autosomal recessive
c. Hydrocortisone
Mineralo corticoids
Sodium supplements 1–3 g
Surgical correction.

A 6:

a. Dysproportionate dwarfism
b. 160 cm.
c. Achondroplasia, cretinism, short limb dwarfism
d. 1.1:1
e. Arachnodactyl, chondrodystrophy, spinal deformity and eunuchoidism.

A 7:

a. Hypoparathyroidism
b. Both low
c. Type I polyendocrinopathy (with Addison's)
d. Basal ganglia calcification.

A 8:

a. 28.92 kg/sq.m, 85th to 94th percentile: "at risk for overweight"
b. Acanthosis nigricans, glucose tolerance test
c. Tibia vara (Blount disease), slipped capital femoral epiphysis, genu valgum.

A 9:

a. Complete androgen insensitivity syndrome
b. 46 XY
c. Testosterone levels. HCG stimulation test with FSH, LH; high testosterone with elevated LH
d. Yes; gonadal malignancy.

A 10:

a. GBS/Ac intermittent porphyria/hypokalemia
b. Ac. intermittent porphyria
c. Urine for porphyrins
d. Glucose/hemin.

A 11:

a. Vitamin D dependent rickets type II (calcitriol resistance)
b. Alopecia
c. Calcitriol in high doses (12.5–20 mcg/d)
d. Periodic serum Ca, P, ALP and urinary Ca excretion.

A 12:

a. Target height in girls: Mid parental height—6.5 cm.

$$\text{Mid parental height} = \frac{\text{Father height} + \text{Mother height}}{2}$$

b. Hemogram with ESR, blood gas, LFT/RFT, stool and urine R/E, bone age, thyroid profile, celiac serology, USG abdomen
c. No growth hormone is required at this time
d. Fine facial features, truncal obesity, central incisor, midfacial anomalies (cleft lip, cleft palate).

A 13:

a. 1.66: 1. Expected at three years of age: 1.3:1
b. Achondroplasia
c. Trident hand with short fingers
d. Short and round iliac bones, flat superior acetabular roof.

A 14:

a. Total insulin dose: $13 \times 0.7 = 9$ units/day.
    A-combination of regular and lente (1:2) insulin subcutaneously in 24 hours.
    2/3 before breakfast and 1/3 before lunch.
    2/3 of 10 = 6 U before breakfast, 3U before lunch.
    Before breakfast: 2/3, i.e. 4U given as lente and 2 U as regular.
    Before lunch 2/3, i.e. 2 U lente and 1 U regular.
b. Counsel for hypoglycemia and its treatment.
c. Glycemic index is a measure of rise of blood sugar after a particular type of food is eaten in comparison with glucose which is 100.
d. Base line investigations-fundus examination, serum lipid profile, thyroid function tests, KFT.

A 15:

a. Mixed metabolic and respiratory acidosis.
b. Expected CO_2 level for the given HCO_3.
    = $HCO_3 \times 1.5 + 8 \pm 2 = 12 \times 1.5 + 8 \pm 2 = 24$–28 mmHg.
c. Anion gap = $(Na) - (Cl + HCO_3) = 136\text{-}115 = 21$.
d. Lactic acidosis (shock, severe anemia, hypoxemia), diabetic ketoacidosis, starvation, alcoholic ketoacidosis, renal failure, inborn errors of metabolism, poisoning with methanol, salicylate.

A 16:

a. McCune-Albright syndrome.
b. Serum levels of estradiol (elevated), luteinizing hormone (low), and follicle stimulating hormone (low).
c. Autonomous activation of gonads.
d. Autonomous hyperactivity of other glands like anterior pituitary adrenals, thyroid, parathyroids, phosphaturia, rickets, hepatic and cardiac involvement, fibrous dysplasia of skeletal system.

A 17:

a. Central precocious puberty.
b. Hypothalamic hamartoma.
c. GnRH stimulation test and MRI brain.
d. GnRH agonists.

A 18:

a. Diabetic ketoacidosis.
b. (i) iv normal saline.
c. (i, iii, iv)—blood gas, serum insulin and serum electrolytes.
d. Cerebral edema.

A 19:

a. Somogyi phenomenon due to production of counter regulatory hormones in the night due to hypoglycemia.
b. Increase pre-breakfast lente and decrease pre-dinner lente.
c. When the blood sugar is ≥ 300 or during sick days.

A 20:

Physical finding	Etiology
1. Disproportionate short stature	Achondroplasia
2. Round head, small nose, small genitals, fine scalp hair	Growth hormone deficiency
3. Round face, short 4th metacarpal, mental retardation	Pseudohypoparathyroidism
4. Central obesity, striae, proximal weakness	Cushing syndrome

A 21:

a. Abetalipoproteinemia.
b. Acanthocytes.
c. Retinitis pigmentosa.
d. Autosomal recessive.
e. Friedrich's ataxia.

A 22:

a. Hypothyroidism.
b. Thyroid dysgenesis (aplasia, hypoplasia or ectopic gland).
c. Craniosynostosis and temperament problems.

A 23:

a. Central precocious puberty-most likely with an identifiable CNS lesion.
b. Acceleration in linear growth, increased testicular volume in the patient.
c. Bone age, T4 and TSH, testosterone, LHRH stimulation test, head MRI.

A 24:

a. 16 years.
b. Craniopharyngioma.
c. Primary gonadal failure.
d. SMR 4 (90%) SMR 5(100%).
e. Imperforate hymen/hematocolpos.
f. Anorexia nervosa.

A 25:

a. Emotional disturbances with motor hyperactivity/irritability/emotional lability.
b. Cardiomegaly and failure, atrial fibrillation, mitral regurgitation due to papillary muscle dysfunction.
c. Propylthiouracil and methimazole.
   Severe reactions: Agranulocytosis, hepatic failure, glomerulonephritis and vasculitis.

A 26:

a. Urea cycle defect.
b.　i. Carbamyl phosphate synthetase (CPS).
　　ii. Ornithine transcarbamylase (OTC).
　　iii. Argininosuccinate synthetase (AS).
　　iv. Argininosuccinate lyase (AL).
　　v. Arginase.
　　vi. N-acetylglutamate synthetase.
c.　i. Sodium benzoate.
　　ii. Phenylacetate.
　　iii. Arginine.
　　iv. Lactulose.
　　v. Neomycin.
　　vi. Citruline.
　　vii. Carnitine.
d. OTC deficiency.
e. OTC defects.

A 27:

a. Biochemical rickets.
b. Renal tubular acidosis.
c. Urine pH, urine anion gap and X-rays of wrist (left usually) for radiological evidence.
d. Treatment for RTA (bicarbonate replacement) and vitamin D (~400 IU/day) along with calcium.

A 28:

a. Acrodermatitis enteropathica.
b. Autosomal recessive.
c. Plasma zinc levels—low levels.
d. 25–50 mg of elemental zinc/day in 2–3 divided doses and Zn rich diet once the supplementation is stopped.

A 29:

Age	Upper: lower segment
Birth	1.7:1
1 year	1.6-1.5:1
3 years	1.3:1
5 years	1.1:1
10 years	0.98:1

A 30:

Findings	Diagnosis
1. Height age = bone age > chronological age	Simple virilizing Congenital adrenal hyperplasia
2. Height age = bone age < chronological age	Familial short stature
3. Height age < bone age = chronological age	Constitutional delay in growth
4. Height age < bone age < chronological age	Growth hormone deficiency

A 31:

a. Nephrogenic diabetes insipidus.

b. $(2 \times Na) + (BUN\ mg/dL/2.8) + (glucose\ mg/dL/18)$
   $= 312 + 5 + 6 = 323\ mOsmol/L.$

c. Hydrochlorthiazide, amiloride, indomethacin, potassium supplementation.

Chapter

5

Genetics

Q1.

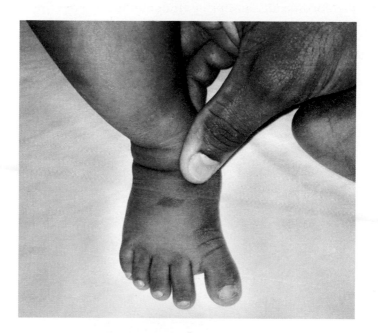

a. What is the finding?
b. What is the commonest condition associated with above finding?
c. Can this be a common variant (Yes/No?)
d. Enlist 1 antenatal cause it can be associated with.

Q2. For each of the conditions below, choose the most closely associated findings from the list above.

a. Tongue fasciculation
b. Gower sign
c. Heliotrope sign
d. Nonthrombocytopenic purpura
e. Thrombocytopenic purpura
    i. Down Syndrome
    ii. Williams syndrome
    iii. Marfan syndrome
    iv. Turner syndrome
    v. Noonan syndrome

Q3.

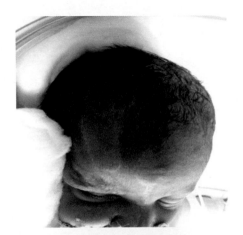

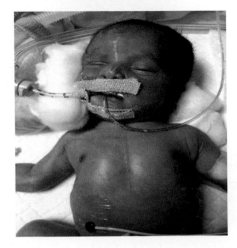

a. What is the diagnosis?
b. What can be the associated abnormalities?

Q4. Given below is a karotype of a 15 day old child

a. Identify the condition and sex of the child

b. Enlist 3 characteristic features

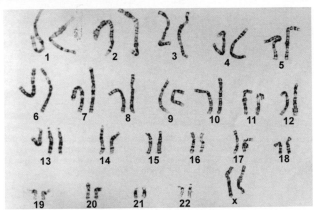

Q5. Enlist the chromosome location and associated cancer in relation to the Gene/oncogene

Gene	Location	Cancer tumour
RBI gene		
APC gene		
WT1gene		
BRCA1 gene		
NF1		
NF2		
Nmyc		
Abl		
Erb-A		
RET		
SIS		

Q6. Study the pedigree chart and answer the questions.

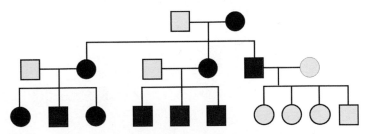

a. Identify the pattern of inheritance in the given pedigree with explanation.

b. Explain the mechanism of this inheritance.

c. Give 2 examples of this pattern of inheritance.

Q7. Study the pedigree chart given below and answer the questions.

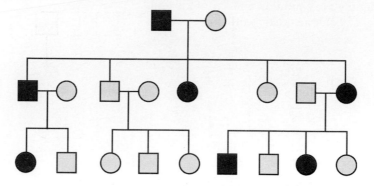

a. What is the pattern of inheritance?
b. Name three conditions with the similar pattern of inheritance.
c. Draw a pedigree chart showing parents with a pair of identical twins.

Q8. Given below is a pedigree chart of a male child with mental retardation.

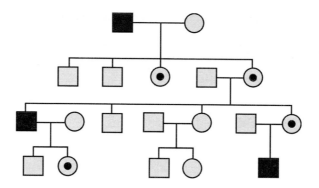

a. Identify the pattern of inheritance.
b. Name three conditions with similar inheritance.
c. What is the risk of getting affected in each pregnancy?

Q9. Identify the degree of consanguinity in the relationships shown with dotted lines in the following pedigree charts.

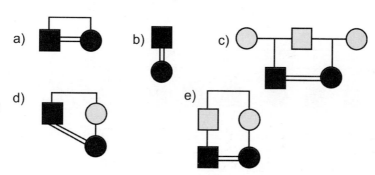

Q10. Study the pedigree chart shown below and answer the questions.

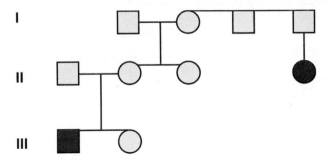

a. Indentify the pattern of inheritance.
b. Give an example of this type of inheritance.
c. If one child of parents with this disorder is already affected, what would be the recurrence risk in the next offspring?
d. It two earlier pregnancies are affected by this disease, what is the recurrence risk in the third offspring?

Q11. A 1-year-old female infant, born of a consanguineous marriage is brought to you with history of developmental delay. Clinically, there is dysmorhism consisting of coarse facies, short stature and corneal clouding. Liver is palpable, 4 cm below costal margin. There is no other family history of a similarly affected child. You make a clinical diagnosis of Hurler syndrome.

a. What features suggest that the diagnosis is Hurler and not Hunter syndrome?
b. How will you evaluate this child to support the diagnosis?
c. Name two modalities of treatment for this child.

Q12. Study the pedigree chart and answer the questions.

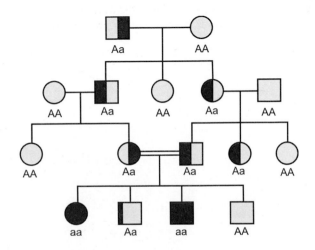

a. What type of inheritance is shown?
b. What is the risk of recurrence in the next pregnancy?
c. Of the following, which is consistent with this type of inheritance?
    i.   Glucose 6 phosphate dehydrogenase deficiency.
    ii. Niemann-Pick disease.
    iii. Meningomyelocele.
    iv. Tuberous sclerosis.

Q13. What is the pattern of inheritance for each of the following.

a. Achondroplasia.
b. Hemophilia B.
c. Congenital adrenal hyperplasia.
d. Glucose 6 phosphate dehydrogenase deficiency
e. Sickle cell disease.
f. Hemophilia A.
g. Phenylketonuria.
h. Duchenne muscular dystrophy.
i. Marfan's syndrome.
j. Huntington's chorea.
k. Neurofibromatosis.

Q14. What do the following symbols represent in the pedigree chart?

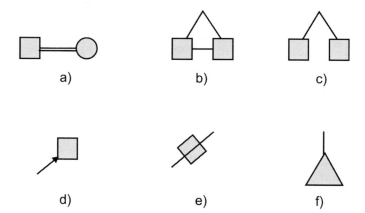

a)   b)   c)

d)   e)   f)

Q15. Study the pedigree chart given below and answer the questions.

a. What is the mode of inheritance?
b. What is the recurrence risk of the disease?
c. Is it possible for the phenotypically normal members of the family to transmit this disease?
d. Which of the following are transmitted in this fashion?
    i.   Noonan's syndrome.
    ii. Galactosemia.
    iii. Diabetes mellitus.
    iv. Hypophosphatemic rickets.

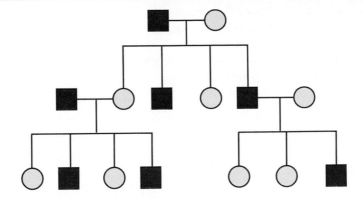

Q16. Full term male neonate was born by normal vaginal delivery to a 23 year old primigravida mother and was noted to have dysmorphic features as mentioned below.

- **Prominent occiput.**
- **Head circumference 29 cm.**
- **Clenched fist with overlapping 3rd and 4th fingers.**
- **Rocker bottom feet.**
a. What is the most probable diagnosis?
b. What is the likely chromosomal configuration of this neonate?
c. Name two congenital heart diseases commonly associated with this syndrome.

Q17. This female child was brought for evaluation of dysmorphic features.

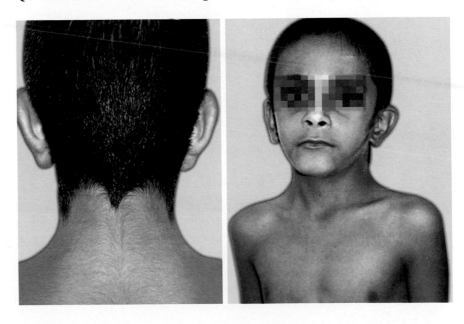

a. What is the most probable diagnosis?
b. Name one cardiac and one renal malformation associated most commonly with this condition.
c. What drug therapy can be provided to these patients?
d. Name one easy OPD procedure to reach a diagnosis.
e. What is the male version of this disease?

Q18. A 32-year-old pregnant lady is at 20 weeks of gestation. She is referred with a positive triple test result.

a. What are the components of triple test, what constitutes an abnormal test and which disease do they screen for?
b. Name three radiological findings that suggest the presence of the disease.
c. How can a definitive diagnosis that can be offered at this stage?

Q19. Study the karyotype of a male neonate born to a 26-year-old primigravida mother with an uneventful antenatal history.

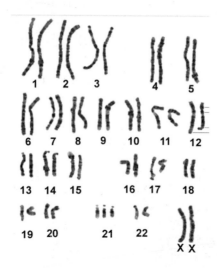

a. The recurrence risk of the condition in the next pregnancy is _____%.
b. If the father is a translocation carrier, the recurrence risk in the next pregnancy is _____%.
c. _____% of these cases occur due to non-disjunction.

Q20. A 14-year-old boy is brought with history of poor scholastic performance, poor social interaction with family and peers and hyperactive behavior. Clinically, he has large ears, a prominent jaw and testicular volume of 36 cc bilaterally. IQ testing shows his IQ to be 75.

a. What is the most probable diagnosis?
b. What is the diagnostic test for the condition?
c. Name the chromosomal site affected in this individual.

Q21. Match the following.

a. Malformation sequence   1. Mechanical (uterine) forces that alter
                               the structure of intrinsically normal tissue

b. Deformation sequence   2. Poor organization of cells into tissues or
                               organs

c. Disruption sequence   3. Single, local tissue morphogenesis
                               abnormality that produces a chain of
                               subsequent defects

d. Dysplasia sequence   4. In utero tissue destruction after a period
                               of normal morphogenesis

Q22. Match the following:

a. Syndrome   Pierre Robin
b. Sequence   VACTERL
c. Association   Trisomy 21

Q23. A 15-year-old male child was brought to pediatric OPD for evaluation of small testes and underdeveloped secondary sex characters. On detailed physical examination, he was found to have prominent breasts bilaterally. He was suspected to have some chromosomal anomaly and a karyotype was done, as shown below.

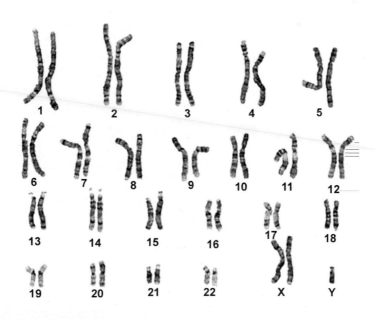

a. What is your diagnosis?
b. Give three salient features of this syndrome.
c. What is the effect on stature in this condition?

Q24. A lady has come to the OPD. Her husband has hemophilia A. There is no history of hemophilia in her family. She is now pregnant and wants genetic counseling. Answer the following questions.

a.   Is her son at a risk for hemophilia?
b.   Her daughter marries a normal man. What are the chances of hemophilia occurring in their children?
c.   How will you offer prenatal diagnosis for hemophilia in the first trimester?

Q25. Answer the questions regarding Turner's syndrome.

a.   What is the characteristic physical external neonatal manifestation?
b.   Name 2 characteristic cardiac anomalies in Turner's syndrome.
c.   Name 2 endocrine problems in Turner's syndrome.
d.   Which GI problems can occur?
e.   Name 3 hormones used in treatment of Turner's syndrome.
f.   What are the most common skeletal abnormalities?

Q26. Answer the following questions with regard to a 5 year old male child with Downs syndrome and mental retardation.

a.   Which one joint will you prefer to examine the most and why?
b.   What would you like to test as a treatable cause for his mental retardation?
c.   Name two blood test you would like do on periodic follow up and why?
d.   Elaborate-46, XY, t (4:8) (p21;q22)

Q27. A 2-year-old girl is brought to the clinic with headache, vomiting, and pallor. Her blood pressure is 130/80 mm Hg. On physical examination, she is noted to have aniridia and a large abdominal mass. Abdominal scanning reveals a poorly vascularized tumor in the upper pole of the right kidney.

a.   What is your most likely diagnosis?
b.   What is the chromosomal defect seen in this condition?
c.   What other abnormalities are associated with this condition?
d.   Name 2 other syndromes associated with Wilm's tumor.

Q28. Study the photograph of this child whose X-ray of one hand is given along with.

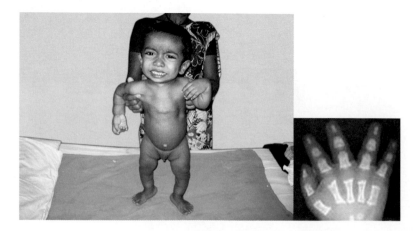

a. What is your likely diagnosis?
b. What inheritance pattern does this disease follows?
c. What is the average IQ in these children?
d. What complications of the vertebral column are likely to occur in this condition?
e. What is this characteristic shortening of limbs called?
f. Where is the abnormal gene in this condition located?

Q29. Match the following.

a.	Germline mosaicism	Some individuals manifest the gene mildly and some severly
b.	Reduced penetrance	Development of more severe expression of the disease through successive generations
c.	Variable expression	Mutation that affects all or some of the germ cells of one parent.
d.	Anticipation	Genetic picture is confused because the apparent father is not the biological father
e.	Non paternity	Some individuals who have inherited the disease do not manifest it phenotypically

Q30. Match the following.

	Disease	Repeat (abnormal) sequence
a.	Myotonic dystrophy	GAA
b.	Friedrich's ataxia	CGG
c.	Fragile X syndrome	CTG
d.	Huntington's disease	CAG

Q31. Given below is a karyotype of a 1-month-old child who presented with characteristic sound produced during crying.

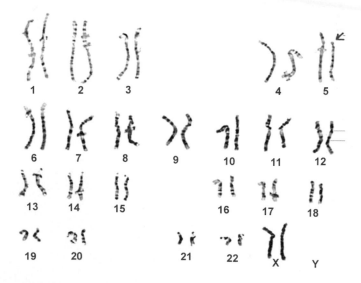

a. Identify the condition and the sex of the child.
b. What is the characteristic presentation in a neonate?
c. What is the life expectancy in this condition?
d. What is the chromosomal defect in this condition?
e. What is the origin of the abnormal chromosome in this condition?

Q32. This male child aged 10 months has been brought with a large tongue. He was born weighing 4.2 kg and had no perinatal or subsequent complication.

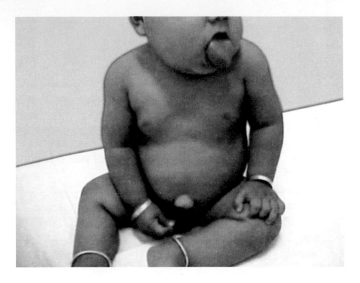

a. What is the most probable diagnosis?
b. What are the components of this syndrome?
c. Which chromosome carries the gene responsible for this disorder?
d. What complications do you expect in such a child?

ANSWERS

A 1:

a. Saddle Gap
b. Trisomy 21
c. Yes
d. Deforming due to an amniotic band.

A 2:

a. 1
b. 3
c. 2
d. 4
e. 5.

A 3:

a. Linear nevus sebaceous syndrome
b.

Central nervous system (brain neoplasms, hemimegalencephaly and lateral ventricle enlargement)
Cardiovascular (aortic coarctation)
Skeletal (localized cranial fibrous dysplasia, skeletal hypoplasia, formation of bony structures, scoliosis and kyphoscoliosis, vitamin D-resistant rickets and hypophosphatemia)
Ophthalmologic (strabismus, retinal anomalies, coloboma, cataracts, corneal vascularization, and ocular hemangiomas) and
Urogenital (horseshoe kidney) systems.

A 4:

a. Triromy 13 Female
b.

General	Low birth weight, single umbilical artery.
CNS	Holoprosencephaly with varying degrees of incomplete fore-brain development. Seizures, severe mental retardation.
Craniofacial	Wide fontanelles, microphthalmia, colobomas, retinal dysplasia cleft\lip and /or cleft palate. Abnormal low-set ears.
Skin	Parietooccipital scalp defects.
Hand and feet	Simian crease, polydactyly.
Cardic	(80%) VSD, PDA, ASD.
Genitalia	Cryptorchidism (male), bicornuate uterus (female).

Most of these children's die within first month (around 80%). Recurrence risk is small unless one of the parent has a balanced translocation.

A 5:

Gene	Location	Cancer tumor
RBI gene	13 (13q14)	Retinoblastoma, osteosarcoma
APC gene	5(q21)	Familial adenomatous polyposis
WT1gene	11(p13)	Wilms tumour
BRCA1 gene	17(q21)	Familial breast and ovarian cancer
NF1	17(q11)	Neurofibromatosis type 1
NF2	22(q12)	Neurofibromatosis type 2
Nmyc	2(p24)	Neuroblastoma
Abl	9(q34)	ALL, CML
Erb-A	17(q11)	Promyelocytic leukaemaia
RET	10(q)	MEN, medullary thyroid carcinoma (germline mutation)
SIS	22(q12)	Glioma

A 6:

a. Mitochondrial inheritance. All affected females have offspring who suffer from the disease. Affected males do not transmit the disease.
b. Mitochondrial DNA present in the ovum transmits the characteristics to the offspring. Such DNA is not present in the sperm.
c. Leigh disease and MELAS (Mitochondrial encephalopathy with lactic acidosis and stroke like syndromes).

A 7:

a. Autosomal dominant.
b. Neurofibromatosis type 1, polycystic kidney disease, tuberous sclerosis, hereditary spherocytosis, Marfans syndrome, osteogenesis imperfecta.
c.

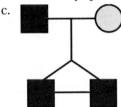

A 8:

a. X-linked recessive.
b. Hemophilia, color blindness, G6PD deficiency, Duchenne muscular dystrophy, Menkes kinky hair disease, adrenoleukodystrophy.
c. The risk is 50% for male child in each pregnancy.

A 9:

a. First degree—sibs from same parents.
b. First degree—parent-child.
c. Second degree—uncle/aunt-niece/nephew.
d. Second degree—half sibs (from different mothers).
e. Third degree-first cousins—children of brother and sister.

A 10:

a. Multifactorial inheritance.
b. Neural tube defect, pyloric stenosis, cleft lip/palate.
c. 3–4%.
d. 10%.

A 11:

a. Hunters syndrome affects males, being X-linked recessive. There is no corneal clouding.
b. X-ray for dysostosis multiplex, urine screening for MPS, enzyme analysis of alpha iduronidase in blood, mutation analysis.
c. Enzyme replacement therapy with alpha iduronidase, bone marrow transplant.

A 12:

a. Autosomal recessive.
b. 25%.
c. (ii) Niemann-Pick disease.

A 13:

a. Autosomal dominant.
b. X-linked recessive.
c. Autosomal recessive.
d. X-linked recessive.
e. Autosomal recessive.
f. X-linked recessive.
g. Autosomal recessive.
h. X-linked recessive.
i. Autosomal dominant.
j. Autosomal dominant.
k. Autosomal dominant.

A 14:

a. Second degree consanguinity.
b. Monozygotic twins.
c. Dizygotic twins.
d. Proband.
e. Stillbirth.
f. Miscarriage.

A 15:

a. Autosomal dominant.
b. 50%
c. No.
d. (i) Noonan syndrome.

A 16:

a. Edward syndrome, trisomy 18.
b. 47 XY + 18.
c. Ventricular septal defect, patent ductus arteriosus.

A 17:

a. Turner syndrome.
b. Bicuspid aortic valve, coarctation of aorta/horse shoe kidney.
c. Growth hormone and estrogens.
d. Buccal smear for barr body.
e. Noonan syndrome.

A 18:

a. Maternal serum alpha fetoprotein (low), unconjugated estradiol (high), free beta hCG (high). They are used to screen for fetal chromosomal anomalies.
b. Second trimester: Increased nuchal fold thickness, short femur, short humerus length, duodenal atresia. First trimester: nuchal fold thickness, nasal bone evaluation.
c. Fetal karyotype by amniocentesis.

A 19:

a. 1%
b. 4–5%
c. 95%

A 20:

a. Fragile X syndrome.
b. Karyotype, DNA studies for fragile X.
c. Xq27.3.

A 21:

a. Malformation sequence	Single, local tissue morphogenesis abnormality that produces a chain of subsequent defects
b. Deformation sequence	Mechanical (uterine) forces that alter the structure of intrinsically normal tissue
c. Disruption sequence	*In utero* tissue destruction after a period of normal morphogenesis
d. Dysplasia sequence	Poor organization of cells into tissues or organs

A 22:

a. Syndrome	Trisomy 21
b. Sequence	Pierre Robin
c. Association	VACTERL

a. A pattern of multiple abnormalities that are related by pathophysiology and result from a common, defined etiology. Trisomy 21, fetal hydantoin syndrome.
b. Multiple malformations that are caused by a single event. Pierre Robin sequence.
c. Non-random collection of malformations where there is unclear relationship amongst the malformations so that they do not fit criteria for a syndrome or sequence VACTERL.

A 23:

a. Klinefelter syndrome.
b. Hypogenitalism, hypogonadism, infertility, tall stature, mental retardation and behavior concerns.
c. Aggressive behavior, antisocial acts, learning difficulties, anxiety.
d. Tall stature with decreased upper to lower segment ratio.

A 24:

a. No.
b. Her male children have a 50% risk of hemophilia.
c. Chorionic villus sampling and detection of the mutation in the hemophilia gene present in the affected child.

A 25:

a. Oedema of hands, feets and posterior neck.
b. • Bicuspid aortic valve
   • Coarctation of aorta
   • Aortic stenosis
   • Mitral valve prolapse
   • Anomalous pulmonary venous drainage.
c. Autoimmune thyroid disease and type 2 diabetes mellitus.
d. Celiac disease; GI bleed and delayed gastric emptying.
e. • GH
   • Estrogen
   • Progesterone
   • Thyroxine (if thyroid dysfunction is present).
f. • Shortening of 4th metatarsal and metacarpal bone
   • Epiphyseal dysgenesis in the joints of knees and elbows
   • Madelung deformity
   • Scoliosis
   • Osseous mineralization
   • Coxa valga.

A 26:

a. Atlantoaxial joint as instable joint (ADI >10 mm) caries a significant risk of neurological injury.
b. Hypothyroidism (T3, T4 and TSH).
c. CBC with peripheral smear- for possibility of leukemia T3,T4,TSH- for possibility of hypothyroidism.
d. 46-Total no. of chromosome:
   XY-Genetic male
   t-Reciprocal translocation
   First parenthesis—Numbers of chromosomes
   Second parenthesis—Bands of chromosomes
   p-short arm and q—Long-arm.

A 27:

a. WAGR syndrome.
b. Microdeletion at 11p13.
c. Wilms tumor, aniridia, genitourinary abnormalities (cryptorchidism, streak ovaries, bicornate uterus, ambiguous genitalia), and mental retardation.
d. Denys-Drash syndrome and Beckwith-Wiedemann syndrome.

A 28:

a. Achondroplasia.
b. Autosomal dominant trait.
c. Normal IQ in these patients.
d. In infancy—stenosis at foramen magnum leading to decreased tone, quadriparesis, apnea and SIDS.
   In childhood—stenosis at L_{1-5} leading to paresthesias, claudication, loss of bladder and bowel control.
e. The patients have a disproportionate short stature—with a normal trunk, short arms and short legs. There is proximal shortening of the limbs (rhizomelic dwarfism).
f. Chromosome 4.

A 29:

a. *Germline mosaicism:* A mutation that affects all or some of the germ cells of one parent. Thus a condition that may appear as a one off mutation recurs in subsequent siblings.
b. *Reduced penetrance:* Some individuals who have inherited the disease do not manifest it phenotypically. They can transmit the gene to next generation, e.g. retinoblastoma.
c. *Variable expression:* Some individuals manifest the gene mildly and some severly, e.g. tuberous sclerosis.
d. *Anticipation:* This is the development of more severe expression of the disease through successive generations. Seen in diseases having trinucleotide repeats in their genes. The number of repeats increases through generations and thus the severity of disease.
e. *Non paternity:* The genetic picture is confused because the apparent father is not the biological father.

A 30:

Disease	Repeat sequence
a. Myotonic dystrophy	CTG
b. Friedrich's ataxia	GAA
c. Fragile X syndrome	CGG
d. Huntington's disease	CAG

A 31:

a. Cri-du-chat syndrome in a female child
b. Cry like a cat due to abnormal larynx development. Usually have low birth weight and may have respiratory problems. The main features are hypotonia, short stature, microcephaly with protruding metopic suture, moonlike face, hypertelorism, bilateral epicanthic folds, high arched palate, wide and flat nasal bridge, and mental retardation.
c. Most of them have a normal lifespan.
d. Microdeletion at short arm of chromosome 5.
e. In 80% cases the affected chromosome comes from father.

A 32:

a. Beckwith Weidmann syndrome.
b. Omphalocele, macroglossia, microcephaly, visceromegaly, hemi-hypertrophy.
c. 11 (11p15.5).
d. Tumors: Wilm's tumor, hepatoblastoma, gonadoblastoma, adrenal carcinoma, rhabdomyosarcoma.

Gastrointestinal Disorders

QUESTIONS

Q1. Answer the following questions regarding acute abdomen.

a. What is the age of peak incidence of appendicitis?
b. What is the classic triad for intussusception?
c. What laboratory tests are satisfactory as an initial screen in patients with abdominal pain?
d. What is the treatment of choice for intussusception?
e. Name three causes of abdominal pain arising from a gonad in a young girl
f. What is the classic finding on appendicitis?
g. How do you test for peritoneal irritation?

Q2. A 3-year-old infant presented with failure to thrive, recurrent diarrhea, irritability and pain abdomen. On examination, he was found to be wasted with edema and finger clubbing. His tTG ELISA for both IgA and IgG was positive.

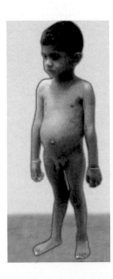

a. What is this condition?
b. Name other serological tests done to diagnose this condition.
c. What will you do to confirm the diagnosis?
d. Name three conditions associated with high frequency of this disease.

Q3. A 15-year-old girl presents to the emergency department with sudden onset of watery diarrhea tinged with blood. The girl was previously healthy. She has been on topical benzoyl peroxide and oral clindamycin for acne vulgaris for past 4 weeks. Physical examination reveals a slightly distended abdomen that is diffusely tender. Her temperature is 38.1°C (100.5°F). She has not been exposed to any uncooked meat and has not eaten any unusual foods.

a. What is the most likely diagnosis?
b. What is the other name for such type of diarrhea?
c. What drugs can be given to cure this? Give the doses and duration of treatment also.

Q4. A mother is being counselled for prevention of allergy. She wants to know which of the following could be (A) food intolerance (B) food hypersensitivity.

  i. Lactose intolerance.
 ii. Urticaria.
iii. Heiner syndrome (cow's milk hypereactivity).
 iv. Celiac disease.
 vi. Irritable Bowel syndrome.

Q5. Match the following.

a. Cow's milk   Paralbumin
b. Egg   Vicilin
c. Peanut   Ovomucoid
d. Fish   Casein

Q6. A 15-month-old chubby male child is admitted with regression of motor milestones since 3 months, rhythmic involuntary movements of (distal > proximal) the upper limbs, tremulous cry and generalized hypotonia. He is having loose stools for the last 7–8 days. He has brownish hair, reticular pigmentation of the skin particularly of the dorsum of the hands . There is pallor and mild hepatosplenomegaly. The involuntary movement stops once patient sleeps.

a. What is your most likely diagnosis?
b. What do you expect in peripheral smear and CT head for this patient?
c. What are the changes in liver if you go for liver biopsy?
d. What is the treatment for involuntary movements?

Q7. DRUG-ORS SALT.

a. Write the composition of WHO ORS in gram per liter.
b. Write the composition of WHO ORS in mmol per liter.
c. In which diarrhea is hypo-osmolar ORS used?

Q8. Study the photograph and answer the following questions.

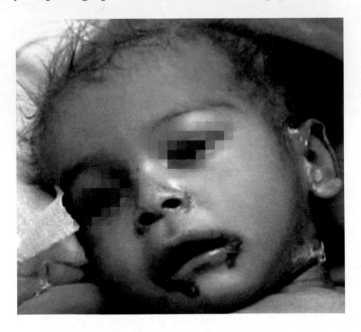

a. Identify this condition which is caused by zinc deficiency.
b. What is the dose of zinc for this condition?
c. Name two other disease where zinc supplements are indicated.

Q9. A 8-month-old girl has been crying and pulling up her legs as if she has abdominal pain. She has vomited several times and is not interested in taking her bottle. She has a fever of 100.5°F. She has not passed stool today. Her parents think that she looks pale and lethargic.

a. Give 2 most likely differential diagnosis.
b. What additional differential diagnosis will you think if this was a male child?

Q10. A 8-year-old girl has periumbilical pain that began 8 hours ago; since then she has vomited once and has had one small, loose, bowel movement. Her last meal was 12 hours ago, and she is not hungry. She denies dysuria and urinary frequency. On examination, she is lying quietly in bed with temperature of 101.5°F. Her other vital signs are normal. Her abdominal examination reveals few bowel sounds, rectus muscle rigidity, and tenderness to palpation, particularly periumbilically. There is some abdominal tenderness with gentle bimanual palpation. She has pain on digital rectal examination. Breath sounds are clear and she has no rashes.

a. What is the most likely diagnosis?
b. What is the single most reliable clinical finding for diagnosing this?
c. What are the sonographic criterias to diagnose this condition?

Q11. A 5-year-old female with severe abdominal pain feels nauseated but has not vomited. She has noticed a faint rash on her feet, legs and buttocks. The temperature is 101°F.

a. What is the most likely diagnosis?
b. What intestinal complications can occur in this condition?
c. What is the medical management for this?

Q12. An 8-month-old female has recent onset of diarrhea. Further history reveals recurrent periods of loose stools, frequent otitis media, and upper respiratory infections. She is being followed for failure to thrive. There has been no vomiting or fever. Her celiac serology and HIV ELISA are negative.

a. What is the most likely condition ?
b. What is its mode of inheritance?
c. Which intestinal protozoal infection is commonly associated with this condition?

Q13. An 18-month-old boy is receiving 'Augmentin' for otitis media. Now he has diarrhea and a diaper rash. There is no fever or vomiting.

a. What is the most likely cause for the diarrhea?
b. Define persistent diarrhea.
c. How do you differentiate between osmotic and secretory diarrhea?

Q14. A marriage dinner was followed by the majority of attendees developing vomiting and watery diarrhea with streaks of blood on the next day. Unaffected attendees did not eat the kheer (milk based sweet). A few ill family members are mildly febrile.

a. What is the most likely etiology for this condition?
b. What is the incubation period of this causative organism?
c. What antibiotics will you prescribe to the affected members?
d. What advice will you give to family members to prevent person-to-person transmission?

Q15. A 12-year-old female has had diarrhea, abdominal pain and flatulence. She often notices some abdominal pain in the late mornings and early afternoon. She has not noticed blood in her stool . The situation worsens on taking milk.

a. What is the likely cause?
b. How do you make a diagnosis in this case?
c. Name 2 conditions where this condition can occur transiently?

Q16. Match the following.

a. Secretory diarrhea   1. Laxative abuse
b. Osmotic diarrhea   2. Irritable bowel disease
c. Increased motility   3. Celiac disease
d. Altered mucosal surface area   4. Cholera
e. Invasiveness   5. Amebiasis

Q17. You are managing a case of persistent diarrhea by taking him to diet plan A (reduced lactose). Three to four days later you are not satisfied with the response and you want to change over to diet B (lactose free).

a. What are the indications for changing diet from A to B or B to C?
b. What are the causes for ineffective ORS therapy while managing a case of acute watery diarrhea ?

Q18. A 2-month-old male, "fussy", baby comes with flatulence, diarrhea and vomiting. He is on breast-feeds. He had viral gastroenteritis 10 days back. Before the infection, mother's milk was well tolerated. Body weight is within normal limits. He is moderately dehydrated. Stool shows presence of reducing sugars with no reaction for glucose. You make a diagnosis of lactose intolerance and start him on reduced lactose diet.

a. What are the indications for changing diet in case of non or poor response?
b. What are diet A, B and C?

Q19. A 2-year-old male child presented with diarrhea of 3 weeks duration with failure to thrive. He was started with nutrition rich feeds (Simyl-MCT drops, HMF sachet and pediasure powder) and antibiotics at a peripheral health center 7 days back. Since then diarrhoea has increased and patient is losing weight. He was moderately dehydrated at admission. His daily stool output is around 185 ml and his stool Na^+ is 42 mEq/L and K^+ is 3.8 mEq/L. His stool was not yet examined for pH and reducing substance.

a. What is the diagnosis based on these investigations?
b. Calculate the osmotic gap.
c. What is the next line of management for this child?

Q20. An 18-month-old male infant manifests failure to thrive, poor appetite, abdominal distension, diarrhea and irritability. He has been well till 9 months of age. Thereafter, he was weaned from breast milk to regular foods. He was diagnosed as a case of celiac disease and started on gluten free diet and was symptom free since then. 3 days back parents had gone for a marriage party and there they fed something to the child. 24 hours later, this child started having protracted vomiting, abdominal distension and was brought to casualty in very sick general condition in shock and had to be ventilated.

a. What is the patient suffering from presently?
b. What is the treatment of choice for this patient (Other than symptomatic support)?
c. Write the conditions in which the celiac disease is more prevalent?

Q21. Answer the following questions.

a. Enlist ingredients, calories/100 mL and protein/100 mL of following diet:
   1. F75
   2. F100
b. What are the time frames for initial treatment, rehabilitation and follow up for the management of severe malnutrition?

Q22. A 10-years-old girl known to have cystic fibrosis presents with a 4 day history of increasing abdominal pain and vomiting which on the last two occasions had contained bile. On examination she has a distended abdomen with palpable loops of bowel. There is also some tenderness in the left iliac fossa but no guarding. Plain abdominal films show dilated bowel loops with fluid levels.

a. Give 2 possible diagnosis.
b. Give one investigation which might help to make a diagnosis.
c. Mention 2 neonatal GI complications of cystic fibrosis.
d. How is cystic fibrosis inherited?

Q23. A 11-year-old girl with cystic fibrosis (CF) is found to be pale on routine general examination. On systemic examination, presence of enlarged liver and spleen is noted. She is investigated and found to have Hb-9 g/dL, TLC 2,000/cumm and platelet count of 56,000/cumm. Liver enzymes are moderately raised.

a. What complication of CF has this girl developed?
b. What is the likely cause for this thrombocytopenia ?
c. What proportion of patients affected with CF develop this complication?

Q24. State TRUE/ FALSE with regards to infant nutrition.

a. Bottle fed infants put weight on a faster rate than breast fed infants.
b. Breast fed infants spend less time in REM sleep than bottle fed infants.
c. Breast and formula milk fed infants have identical amino acid profiles.
d. Breast milk and formula milk contain identical quantities of PUFA.

Q25. An 8-month-old infant is admitted with one day history of persistent crying and not taking his feeds. Crying is episodic and is associated with leg and hip flexion. On abdominal examination, a centrally placed 'sausage-shaped' mass is palpable.

a. Give the most likely diagnosis.
b. What finding is noted on rectal examination of this child?
c. What relevant investigation would you like to do for this child?
d. What would be the diagnosis if, in addition to the above, the infant was lethargic and pale with abdominal tenderness and absent bowel sounds?
e. What would be the next two steps in management in order of priority?

Q26. A 4-week-old male baby presents with a history of vomiting for 3 days. Despite this, he is eager to feed. On examination there is dehydration but no fever. His investigations are shown below.

Na^+—128 mEq/L ; K^+—3.0 mEq/L; Cl^- —86 mEq/L ; HCO_3—36 mmol/L; pH 7.50.

a. Describe these results.
b. Give 3 differential diagnoses for this condition.
c. What is the most likely diagnosis?
d. Give 3 most useful investigations you will carry out for this child.

Q27. A 12-month-old infant presents with bilious vomiting and abdominal distention for 10 hours. His mother states that the infant has been constipated since birth and failed to pass meconium during the first 48 hours of life. On examination, he is very irritable. His length and weight are both below the 5th percentile according to his age. His abdomen is moderately distended. After a digital rectal examination, a fair amount of stool ejects out from the anus.

a. What is the most likely diagnosis?
b. Give an alternative name for this condition.
c. What are the common conditions associated with this condition?
d. What is the recent treatment strategy used for this condition?

ANSWERS

A 1:

a. Teenage and young adult years (12–18 years); males slightly more than females.
b. Severe episodic pain, "currant jelly" stool, transverse tubular abdominal mass.
c. CBC, BUN, creatinine, electrolytes, blood sugar, urine analysis.
   Serum amylase, lipase, aminotransferase.
   Examination of stool.
   Chest X-ray and flat and upright film of abdomen.
d. Hydrostatic reduction. However in patients with prolonged intussusception with signs of shock, peritoneal irritation, intestinal perforation or pneumatosis intestinalis, reduction should not be attempted.
e. Ovarian tumor, torsion of an ovary, ruptured ovarian cyst.
f. Right lower quadrant tenderness.
g. Rebound tenderness.

A 2:

a. Celiac disease.
b. Antigliadin and antiendomyseal antibodies.
c. Small bowel biopsy.
d. Down's syndrome, Turner's syndrome, William's syndrome, thyroiditis, selective IgA deficiency.

A 3:

a. Pseudomembranous enterocolitis.
   (It is caused by the toxins produced by *Clostridium difficile*. It occurs in some patients after treatment with antibiotics (especially clindamycin, cephalosporins, and amoxicillin). Patients develop fever and abdominal pain with diarrhea containing leukocytes and blood).
b. Antibiotic associated diarrhea.
c. Most essential step is to discontinue the current antibiotic, if possible.
   Oral metronidazole 20–40 mg/kg/day q 6-8 hourly for 7–10 days.
   Intravenous vancomycin 25–40 mg/kg/day q 6 hourly for 7–10 days.

A 4:

  i. A
 ii. B
iii. B
 iv. B
  v. A

A 5:

a. Cow's milk   Casein
b. Egg   Ovomucoid
c. Peanut   Vicilin
d. Fish   Paralbumin

A 6:

a. Nutritional tremor syndrome.
b. P/S—megaloblastic anemia; CT head—cerebral atrophy.
c. Liver biopsy—fatty changes.
d. Carbamazepine and propranolol.

A 7:

a. NaCl   = 3.5 g/L
    KCl   = 1.5 g/L
    $NaHCO_3$ = 2.5 g/L
    Glucose   = 20 g/L
b. Na^+ = 90 mEq/L
    K^+ = 20 meq/L
    Cl^- = 80 mEq/L
    Glucose   = 111 mmol/L
    Citrate   = 10 mEq/L
c. Rotavirus induced diarrhea

A 8:

a. Acrodermatitis enteropathica.
b. 50–150 mg/day.
c. Acute or persistent diarrhea, Wilson's disease.

A 9:

a. Intussusception, gastroenteritis, obstructed hernia.
b. Testicular torsion.

A 10:

a. Acute appendicitis.
b. Localized abdominal tenderness is the single most reliable finding in the diagnosis.
c. The ultrasound criteria for appendicitis include:
    • Wall thickness <6 mm
    • Luminal distention
    • Lack of compressibility
    • Complex mass in the right lower quadrant
    • Fecalith.

Findings suggestive of advanced appendicitis on ultrasound include:
    • Asymmetric wall thickening.
    • Abscess formation.
    • Associated free intraperitoneal fluid.
    • Surrounding tissue edema.
    • Decreased local tenderness to compression.

A 11:

a. Anaphylactoid purpura.
b. Hemorrhage, obstruction, intussusception.

c. Therapy with oral or intravenous corticosteroids (1–2 mg/kg/day) is often associated with improvement of both gastrointestinal and CNS complications.

A 12:

a. IgA deficiency.
b. Autosomal dominant with variable expression.
c. Intestinal giardiasis.

A 13:

a. Antibiotic induced diarrhea due to 'Augmentin'.
b. Diarrhea persisting for 14 days or beyond and associated with malnutrition.
c. Diarrhea.

	Osmotic	Secretory
• Volume of stool	< 200 mL/24 h	>200 mL/24 h
• Response to fasting	Diarrhea stops	Diarrhea continues
• Stool Na$^+$	<70 mEq/L	>70 mEq/L
• Reducing substances	Positive	Negative
• Stool pH	<5	>6

A 14:

a. *Salmonella* food poisoning.
b. 6–72 hours (mean 24 hours).
c. Antibiotics are not generally recommended for the treatment of *Salmonella* gastroenteritis because they may suppress normal intestinal flora and prolong the excretion of *Salmonella* and the remote risk for creating the chronic carrier state.
d. Clean water supply and education in hand washing and food preparation and storage is critical in reducing person-to-person transmission.

A 15:

a. Lactose intolerance.
b. • Measurement of carbohydrate in the stool, using a clinitest reagent, which identifies reducing substances, is a simple screening test.
   • Acidic stool with reducing substance >2+ suggests carbohydrate malabsorption. (Sucrose or starch in the stool is not recognized as a reducing sugar until after hydrolysis with hydrochloric acid, which converts them to reducing sugars).
   • Breath hydrogen test.
   • Small bowel biopsies can give a confirmatory evidence.
c. Celiac disease and after Rota virus infection.

A 16:

a. Secretory diarrhea   Cholera
b. Osmotic diarrhea   Laxative abuse
c. Increased motility   Irritable bowel disease
d. Altered mucosal surface area   Celiac disease
e. Invasiveness   Amebiasis

A 17:

a. • Stool frequency > 10/day after 48 hrs of starting particular diet.
   • Return of signs of dehydration anytime after starting diet.
   • Failure to establish weight gain by 7th day.
b. • High purge rate (>5 mL/kg/h).
   • Persistent vomiting >3 vomiting/h
   • Ileus or abdominal distension.
   • Incorrect preparation.
   • Glucose malabsorption.

A 18:

a. Indications:
   – Stool frequency >10 watery stool/day even after 48 hours of starting diet.
   – Return of the signs of dehydration any time after staring diet.
   – Failure to establish weight, gain by 7th day of dietary management.
b. Types of diet:
   – Diet A (reduced lactose).
   – Diet B (lactose free).
   – Diet C (Monosaccharide based diet).

A 19:

a. Chronic diarrhea (secondary lactose intolerance—Osmotic diarrhea).
b. Osmotic gap: $290 - (2 \times Stool\ Na^+ + K^+) = 290 - [2 \times (42 + 3.8)] = 198.4$
   If Gap >100 its osmotic diarrhoea.
c. Remove the osmotic load from the diet and stop feeding for 24 hours and then restart with lactose free diet.

A 20:

a. Celiac crises.
b. Systemic steroids.
c. IgA deficiency, Down's syndrome, Turner's syndrome, William syndrome, thyroiditis.

A 21:

a. *F75:* Dried skim milk 25 g, sugar 70 g, cereal flour 35 g, vegetable oil 27 g, mineral mix 20 mL,vitamin mix 140 mg, water to make 1000 mL. Calories 75 kcal, protein 0.9 g.
   F 100: Dried skim milk 80 g, sugar 50 g, vegetable oil 60 g, mineral mix 20 ml, vitamin mix 140 mg, water to make 1000 mL. Calories 100 kcal, protein 2.9 g.
b. Day 1–7 for initial treatment; week 2–6 for rehabilitation and week 7 to 26 for follow-up.

A 22:

a. Distal intestinal obstruction syndrome (DIOS) and intussusception.
b. Abdominal USG or gastrograffin enema.
c. Meconium ileus, meconium plug, meconium peritonitis.
d. Autosomal recessive.

A 23:

a. Hepatic cirrhosis with portal hypertension.
b. Hypersplenism.
c. <10%.

A 24:

a. True   b. True
c. False   d. False

A 25:

a. Intussusception.
b. Blood or bloody mucus.
c. Plain abdominal X-ray, urine and electrolyte evaluation (as dehydration and electrolyte imbalances are common).
d. Peritonitis/intestinal perforation.
e. Fluid replacement followed by open reduction via laparotomy.

A 26:

a. Hypochloraemic, hyponatremic, hypokalemic alkalosis.
b. UTI, GER, CHPS.
c. Congenital hypertrophic pyloric stenosis (CHPS).
d. • TLC/DLC.
    • Test during feeding—palpate the 'pyloric tumour'.
    • Urine for microscopy and culture.

A 27:

a. Hirschsprung disease.
b. Congenital aganglionic megacolon.
c. Hirschsprung disease may be associated with other congenital defects, including:
    i. Down's syndrome.
   ii. Smith-Lemli-Opitz syndrome.
  iii. Waardenburg syndrome.
  iv. Cartilage-hair hypoplasia syndrome.
   v. Congenital hypoventilation ("Ondine curse") syndromes.
  vi. Urogenital or cardiovascular abnormalities.
  vii. Microcephaly and abnormal facies.
viii. Mental retardation.
  ix. Autism.
   x. Cleft palate.
  xi. Hydrocephalus.
  xii. Micrognathia.
d. Laparoscopic endorectal pull-through procedures, are the treatment of choice.

Hematology and Oncology

QUESTIONS

Q1. A 5-year-old child has a massive GI bleed. He weighs 20 kg.

His clotting time is 13 minutes. His PT test is 42 secs, (control 15 secs) and aPTT test is 64 secs, (control is 29).

His Hb is 11 g and platelet count is 2.5 lakhs.

a. What blood product would you transfuse?
b. How much of above transfusion is required?
c. List 4 other indications for transfusion with this blood product.

Q2. 11-year-old girl presents to ED with breathing difficulty since 1 day. She has been admitted with a similar condition 2 years back. This was associated with a bout of hemoptysis back then. She was found to have severe anemia and received 2 units of blood. She has been on iron therapy since due to persistently low Hb.

O/E she is very pale with not much chest findings.

Investigations revealed a Hb of 5, TLC and platelets are normal. Her MCV is 65, RDW is 21 and RBC count is 2 million with low MCH and MCHC.

Chest X-ray shows bilateral infiltrates.

a. What is your diagnosis?
b. What are the various ways to confirm the diagnosis?
c. What is the drug commonly used to treat this?

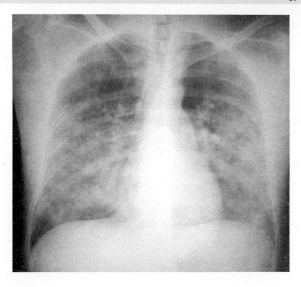

Q3. A 13-year-old girl presents with fever since last 3 months. This is associated with night sweats. She has lost 10 kg weight in last 2 months.

O/E she has supraclavicular node 3 × 3 cm, bilateral submandibular and jugulodigastric node 2 × 2 cm. No organomegaly is present.

Biopsy of the lymph node shows.

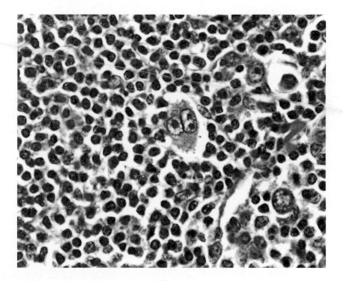

a. What is the diagnosis?
b. What is the classification?
c. What is the staging called?
d. Name 4 drugs commonly used to treat this condition.

Q4. A 2-years-old female child has fever and lymphadenopathy for 3 weeks

- O/E has splenohepatomegaly.
- CBC shows Hb 5, TLC 2000, platelets 24000. No immature cells in the smear.
- Bone marrow shows extensive hemophagocytosis.
- Father says that the previous child died at 1 year of age with a similar illness. She too had a lack of blood formation and bleeding.
    - a. What is the likely diagnosis?
    - b. What are the other biochemical abnormalities that will lead to the diagnosis?
    - c. In non familial state, what infections can precipitate this.

Q5. A 1.5-year-old boy presents with swelling in the right ankle after a trivial fall. He has history of easy bruisisng a prolonged bleeding from injection site. His maternal uncle died of a bleeding disorder.

- a. Name a screening test to clinch the diagnosis.
- b. What does RICE stand for in the management of this disease?
- c. Name the drug used to control bleeding in case he suffers another joint bleed.

Q6. A 6-month-old child is being evaluated for purpura. His low platelet count is 40000/cumm. He has been on various skin ointments for a non-resolving dermatitis. He has been given antibiotics twice for management of otitis media and LRTI.

- a. What is the diagnosis?
- b. Name two screening tests.
- c. What is the treatment?
- d. What are the long term risks?

Q7. A 4-year-old boy presents with fever for 10 days, lethargy, poor oral intake, abdominal distension and decreased urine output. He is sick looking and has diffuse tenderness in his abdomen. USG abdomen reveals multiple lymph nodal masses with hepatosplenomegaly. His CBC is normal with LDH of 12000 and urea of 120 and creat of 2.2. His uric acid is 12.5.

- a. What is the likely diagnosis?
- b. What is the treatment to be initiated at the primary care center?
- c. What is the novel agent used to treat this complication?
- d. What is the characteristic histological appearance of this condition?
- e. What is the overall prognosis of this condition?

Q8. A 17-year-old boy presents with progressive lethargy, loss of appetite.

- **O/E Pallor, ecchymotic spots, no lymphadenopathy or organomegaly, no dysmorphology**
- **Investigations**
    - CBC:
    - Hb 7
    - TLC 5000
    - Platelet count 12000

- DLC: N 10 L 85 E 3 M 2
- MCV 86
- RBC 2.5
- RDW 14
- Peripheral smear: Pancytopenia, No immature cells
- Retic count: 0.4%

The bone marrow picture of this patients shows:

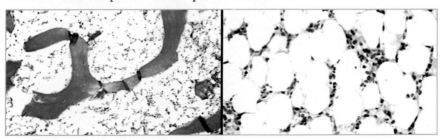

a. What is the diagnosis?
b. What will be 2 important investigations before you embark on treatment?
c. What are the 2 treatment options?

Q9.

a. Name the cell marked by the arrow.
b. Name the dye used to stain the cell.
c. What is the normal value of this cell in a child?
d. Name 2 conditions in which these cells are elevated.

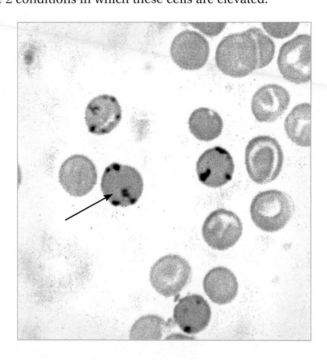

Q10. A 12-year-old male presents with severe pancytopenia. His bone marrow biopsy confirms severe aplastic anemia. He is referred for a BMT to higher center. O/E: he is found to have the following.

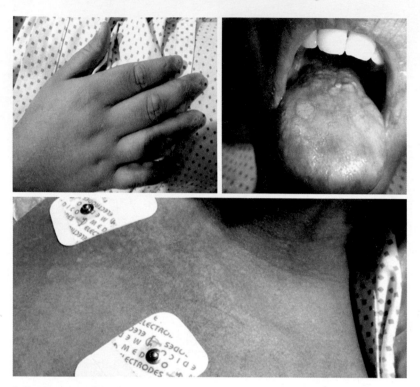

a. What is your diagnosis?
b. What is the basic pathophysiological defect in these patients?
c. How do you treat them?
d. What are other potential lethal complications?

Q11. A 7-year-old male child presents with fever, pallor and ecchymotic spots.

- O/E: pallor+
- Spleen 2 cm BLCM
- Liver 4 cm BRCM
- Testes enlarged
- CBC shows pancytopenia.

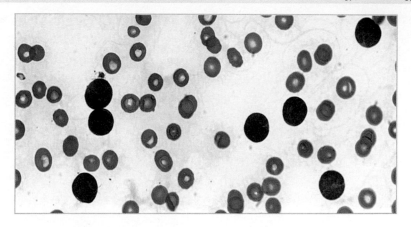

a. What is your diagnosis?
b. How to confirm the diagnosis?
c. Name 3 agents used to treat this?
d. What is the success rate of treatment with modern day regimens?

Q12. A 15-year-old girl with history of generalised weakness and increasing pallor since one month, had history of fever 1 week back. No history of bleeding, loose stools, passage of worms

- Afebrile.
- Pallor ++,
- Petechiae +
- No icterus.
- No significant lymphadenopathy.
- No organomegaly.

Investiations

- Hb-   6.1
- TLC-   5000 ANC low
- Platelets   27,000
- MCV-   102.8
- MCH-   28.6
- MCHC-   32.2
- RDW-   31.2
- Retic count.   2%

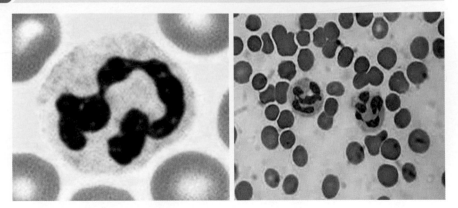

a. Name the cell seen in the smear
b. What is your diagnosis?
c. How do you treat such a patient?

Q13. A 6 years-old-boy being looked after a single mother as father died a year back of a chronic illness, excessive bruising for past 9 months platelets documented to be < 20,000 on many occasions, bone marrow showed megakaryocytic thrombocytopenia. Initially responded to steroids but recurs on tapering of steroids and significant weight loss in last 6 months

Examination
- Bruises both legs
- Mild pallor
- B/L cervical lymph nodes
- Thrush
- Spleen 1 cm palpable.

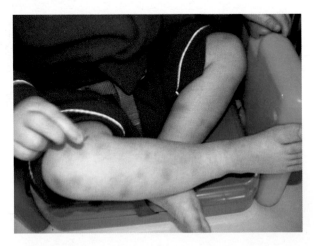

a. What is the most likely diagnosis?
b. What is the investigation of choice?
c. What agents are used to treat this condition?

Q14. 4-year-old boy is under evaluation for mild anemia.

- CBC shows a Hb 9 g% TLC 6000 platelet 2.4 lakhs
- MCV 62
- RBC 5.5
- RDW 13
- PS shows microcytic hypochromic anemia
  a. What is the likely diagnosis?
  b. What will be the test of choice and the expected results?
  c. What treatment will be given to this child?

Q15. A 2-year-old girl presented with fever of 1 month duration, difficulty in walking because of pain, multiple bony swelling on the skull and proptosis.

- O/E she is pale, hypertensive and a diffuse abdominal mass is palpable.

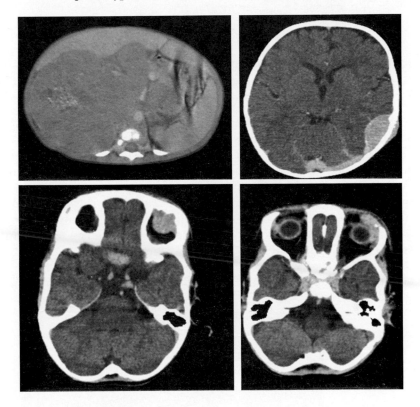

a. What is the likely diagnosis?
b. Name a noninvasive and an invasive test that can lead to a diagnosis.
c. What is the most likely site of origin of the disease?

Q16. A 2-year-old boy presents with a new onset unsteady gait. Mother has noticed roving movements in eyes. Local doctor has done a chest X-ray along with other routine work up which reveals a significant mediastinal shadow.

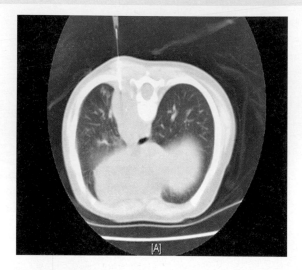

a. What is the likely diagnosis?
b. What is the treatment?
c. What is the prognosis of this condition?

Q17. A 14 year old boy presents with cough for 1 month and difficulty in breathing for last 2 weeks. He was given oral antibiotics after 1 week of illness. A local doctor did a Chest Xray which revealed a significant pleural effusion on the left side and empirically started him on ATT. However his condition worsened and he presented in the emergency with severe respiratory distress orthopnea and stridor. Chest Xray reveals complete opacification of left side. CBC is normal. Pleural fluid analysis reveals some abnormal cells. Scan done after pleural tap reveals a mediastinal mass compressing the trachea.

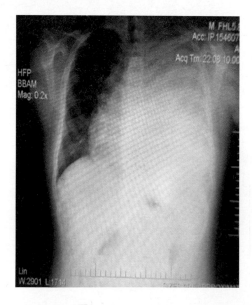

a. What is the most likely diagnosis?
b. What test will most easily clinch the diagnosis?
c. What are the precautions to be taken in this condition?
d. What is the life saving therapy in this condition?

Q18. A 12-year-old boy presents with fever of 2 weeks duration with swellings in the neck. His CBC shows a TLC of 2.9 Lakh/cumm. His serum K and creatinine is 6 and 1.2 respectively.

a. What is the likely diagnosis?
b. What biochemical abnormalities are expected?
c. What management needs to be done before starting definitive therapy?

Q19. A 5-year-old boy presents with pallor and passing dark-colored urine. Three days prior the patient had low-grade fever and dry cough. Initial CBC revealed a hemoglobin level of 4.5 g/dL, a HCT of 14%, a WBC count of 9,100/mm³, (Normal DLC) and a platelet count of 3,72,000/mm³. In the past he has received 2 blood transfusions for fever and acute anemia at 18 months of age. Both parents are thalassemia carriers. Physical examination: Temperature–38.3°C, with marked pallor. CVS–Systolic ejection murmur grade II/VI at left upper sternum. Abdomen–Spleno-hepatomegaly is present. The Hb electrophoresis report is shown.

ANALYTE	ID	%	TIME	AREA
Unknown	1	11.9	0.013	531911
Unknown	2	1.5	0.31	67705
Unknown	3	5.7	0.64	254986
P1		2.1	0.97	92438
F		3.5	1.26	158832
P2		3.7	1.42	164718
P3		3.4	1.78	151986
A0		67.2	2.88	2997869
C-WINDOW		0.9	5.07	38296
		TOTAL AREA		4458732
F		3.5%	A2	0.0%

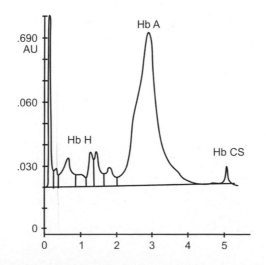

a. What is your diagnosis?
b. What may be the trigger for this crisis?

Q20. A 7-year-old child is admitted for LRTI. This is his 5th episode of severe pneumonia apart from 4 episodes of severe diarrhea in past. On transfusing blood in view of anemia (Hb 5.5 g%), he develops a severe transfusion reaction. He has never received a transfusion in the past and clerical errors of a blood group mismatch are excluded.

a. What immunological defect is most likely present?
b. What would you advise the parents of this child to prevent a recurrence of reaction?

Q21. A 5-year-old male child is recently diagnosed as a case of acute myeloid leukemia. He is clinically stable with a RR of 20/min, normal blood pressure and SpO_2 of 95% in room air. His blood gas is as follows:

pH–7.43; $PaCO_2$–34 mmHg; PaO_2–47.6 mmHg; HCO_3^-–24 mEq/L.

Further investigations show leucocytosis (TLC—60,000/cu mm) and a normal chest X-ray.

a. Analyze the blood gas report.
b. What step will you take to improve PaO_2 in this patient?

Q22. Study the photograph of the peripheral smear provided and answer the questions.

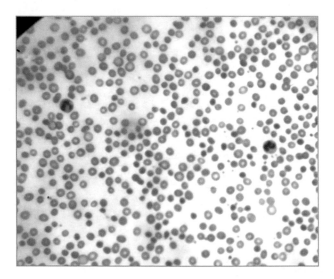

a. What is your diagnosis?
b. What is the drug used to treat this condition?
c. What is the first clinical evidence of improvement after starting the therapy?

Q23. Answer the given questions in relation to methemoglobinemia.

a. At what level of MHg is cyanosis visible?
b. What is the expected pulse oximetry saturation in such a patient?
c. Name the drug used in the treatment of this condition and give its dose
d. In which scenario is this drug contraindicated?
e. Acute methemoglobinemia is characterized by all *except:*
  i. Cyanosis not responding to oxygen.
  ii. Normal cardiopulmonary examination.
  iii. Chocolate color ABG sample.
  iv. Pulse oximetry SpO_2 low with low PaO_2

Q24. A 1½-year-old male child presented with episodes of on and off fast breathing for the past 5 months, occasionally associated with cough . He is also having high-grade intermittent fever for last 2 weeks. Empirical antitubercular treatment for past 3 months has had no benefit. There is a past history of chronic otitis media with perforation and the child has been taken to the dentist twice for loose teeth and swollen gums. On examination, seborrheic dermatitis, pallor and hepatomegaly (5 cm below costal margin) are the salient positive findings.

a. What is your most probable diagnosis?
b. What is the characteristic lesion found on skeletal survey?
c. What do you expect to find in the bone marrow?
d. What is the characteristic electron microscopy finding?

Q25. Study the photomicrograph and answer the question.

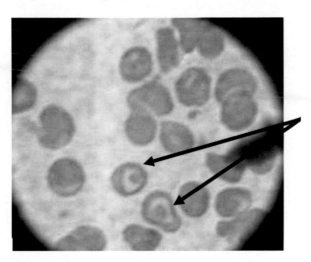

a. Identify the abnormality on peripheral smear.
b. Name 4 conditions where these cells can be seen.

Q26. A 10-year-old girl, with ITP diagnosed since 6 months of age presents with ecchymotic patch on her waist (shown in the photograph) and has uncontrollable epistaxis. Her platelet count is 4000/mm³. Answer the following questions.

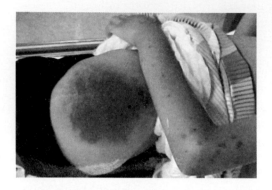

a. Which 3 investigations would you advise in her?
b. What 4 measures either singly or in combination can be used to treat life-threatening hemorrhage in ITP?
c. What is the indication of doing bone marrow examination in a suspected case of ITP?
d. When do you call ITP to be chronic?
e. Give 2 drugs that cause thrombocytopenia.

Q27. This 3-year-old boy develops easy bruising over the body with hematoma formation even with minor trauma.

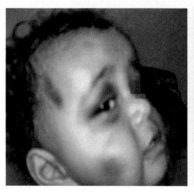 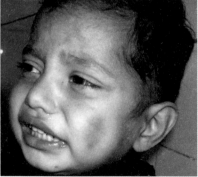

a. What is the most likely diagnosis?
b. Which one investigation would you advice?

c. What is the mode of inheritance?
d. Which type would he be categorized as?

Q28. A 12-year-old boy is tested for sickle cell disease. His father is known to have sickle cell trait. His lab results are as follows: Hb 10.1 g/dL, RBC–6 lacs/cu mm, MCV– 65 fl, MCH–21.1 pg, MCHC–30 g/dl, sickle test positive, HbS–71%, HbA–21.5%, HbA2–4.5%, HbF–3%, Serum ferritin–19 mcg/L.

a. What hemoglobinopathy does the boy have?
b. What hemoglobinopathy do you expect on testing the mother?
c. Which bacterial infections are more common in such patients?

Q29. Match the clinical diagnosis with the hematological findings.

a. Kawasaki disease   1. Splenomegaly in a 6-year-old
b. Alpha thalassemia major   2. Increased fetal Hb
c. Beta thalassemia major   3. Hyposplenism in a 6-year-old
d. Sickle cell disease   4. Thrombocytosis
e. G6PD deficiency   5. Oxidant induced red cell damage
f. Hereditary spherocytosis   6. Hydrops fetalis

Q30. A 4-year-old boy presents with severe pain in both of his legs. On physical examination, his temperature is 37.7°C (99.8 °F), blood pressure is 108/68 mmHg, pulse rate is 96/min, and respirations are 22/min. He is noted to have marked pallor on his lips and palpebral conjunctiva. Numerous purpura and petechiae are noted on his skin. There is bilateral cervical lymphadenopathy. His spleen is palpable 3 cm below his left costal margin. Laboratory evaluation reveals a white blood cell count of 1600/mm³; hemoglobin, 6.1 g/dL; and platelets, 36,000/mm³.

a. What is your most probable diagnosis?
b. What is the peak age incidence of this disease and in which sex is it more common?
c. What is the diagnostic investigation and what do you find?
d. Mention 3 poor prognostic factors for this disease.

Q31. On routine screening of a 12-month-old child, the hemoglobin was found to be 8 gm/dL.

a. What details in a nutritional history would be important?
b. What nutritional intervention might you suggest, besides or in addition to iron supplementation?
c. What specific instructions and plans for follow-up would you give the parents in order to optimize iron supplementation?

Q32. Study the peripheral smear shown below and answer the following questions.

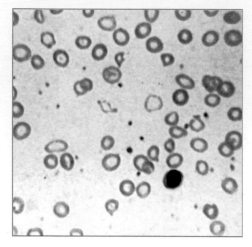

a. Comment on this smear on all the 3 cell lines.
b. Mention at least 3 differentials for this smear.
c. What is the diagnostic test for confirmation?

Q 33. Answer the following questions.

a. What are the 3 classes of histiocytosis syndrome in children?
b. Name 2 features of each in class I histiocytosis.
    i. Dermal manifestations.
    ii. Endocrine problems.
    iii. X-ray skeletal findings.
c. Name three biochemical abnormalities seen in class II histiocytosis.

Q 34. Study the smear shown below and answer the following questions.

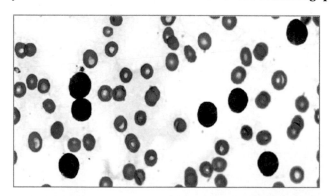

a. What is your diagnosis based on the smear shown above?
b. What other test would you like to do to confirm your diagnosis?
c. What possible differential diagnosis can you think of?
d. Do you need to screen the family if your suspicion comes out positive?
e. Can there be skin involvement in this condition? What is it known as?

Q35. Study the smear shown below and answer the following questions.

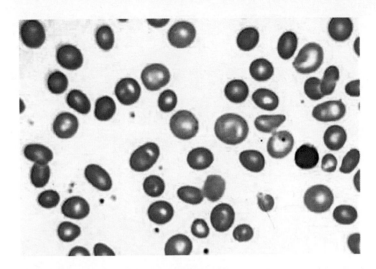

a. Identify the abnormality shown on the peripheral smear above.
b. Name four causes for this condition?
c. Name one drug which can cause this condition?

Q36. Study the smear shown below and answer the given questions.

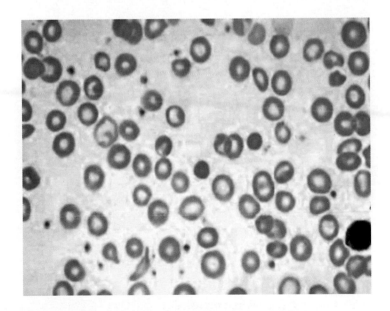

a. Name type of anemia seen on this peripheral smear.
b. Enumerate 4 causes of this type of anemia.
c. What is RDW and RDW is increased in which of these anemias?

Q37. Study the smear below and answer the given questions.

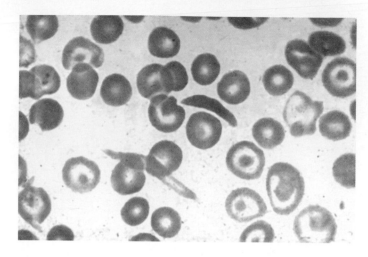

a. What are your findings on this smear?
b. What is the mutational change that leads to this?
c. Which viral infection posseses a unique threat for patients with this disease?

Q38. Study the smear below and answer the given questions.

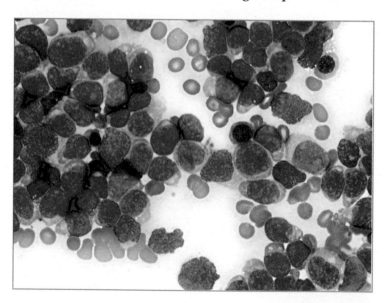

a. What are your findings on this smear?
b. What is your most probable diagnosis?
c. Name four diseases in which this condition can occur.
d. An increased association with which viral infection has been associated with this condition?

Q39. Study the smear below and answer the given questions.

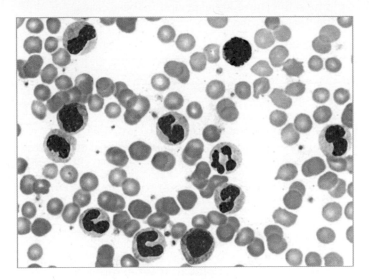

a. What are your findings on this smear?
b. What is the average half-life of neutrophil in circulation?
c. Mention 3 drugs that can cause neutropenia.

Q40. A 3-month-old male child presented with diarrhea and ear discharge from the both ears for the last 15 days. Child is on exclusive breast milk. Since diarrhea he has lost 1 kg weight and his current weight is 3.5 kg. He was given BCG and hepatitis B at birth, BCG left no scar mark. Rest of the history including birth history is normal. On examination, he has mucocutaneous candidiasis and multiple pyaemic abscesses all over the body along with a eczematous rash at abdomen. There is mild hepatosplenomegaly and there are no other findings. His initial investigations revealed lymphopenia (<2000) and low IgA levels. His antibody levels against HBSAg (after 2 doses) are absent. On CT scan examination, he was found to have a very small thymus (< 1 gm) and very underdeveloped tonsils and adenoid tissue.

a. What is the most probable diagnosis?
b. What is the specific treatment, if any?
c. What special precaution should be taken if the infant requires transfusion of a blood product and why?

Q41. A 2-month-old previously healthy full term female infant presents with fever, lethargy and poor feeding for 12 hours. Family history reveals that a male sibling died suddenly at the age of two months, prior to the birth of this child. There is h/o delayed cord fall. Physical examination reveals a lethargic child with RR–70/m, HR–185/m, BP–mean 25 mmHg, T–39.5°C and poor peripheral perfusion. Chest reveals retractions. Abdomen is soft and lab results reveal Hb of 9.8 gm, TLC 65000 (P-90%) and platelet count 1.4 lacs. P/S is normal and no organomegaly.

a. What is the most likely diagnosis?
b. What common infections are expected in these cases?
c. What is the treatment of choice?

Q42. Match the following.

Disease	Deficiencies
a. Lupus-like syndrome	1. C5, 6, 7, 8, 9
b. Recurrent neisserial infections	2. C3
c. Severe recurrent pneumococcal infection	3. C1Q
d. Fatal meningococcal infections in males	4. C1 inhibitor
e. Non-pitting edema	5 Properdin

Q43. Answer the following questions on thrombotic thrombocytopenic purpura (TTP).

a. Give the characteristic pentad of TTP.
b. What is the etiology of familial TTP?
c. What treatment strategy is most suitable for TTP?
d. What cells do you see on peripheral smear in this case?

Q44. A bone marrow aspirate of a 18-month-old child with features of delayed milestones, muscle hypertonia, recurrent aspiration pneumonia and hepatosplenomegaly is shown above.

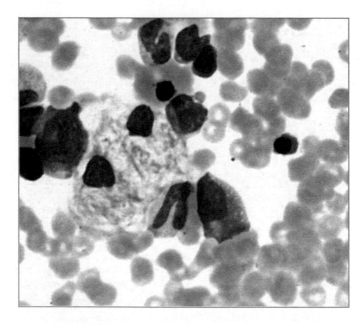

a. Describe the findings seen on the smear.
b. Give 2 clinical differential diagnoses for this.
c. What management strategy is advised in such a case?

Q45. Study the smear shown below and answer the given questions.

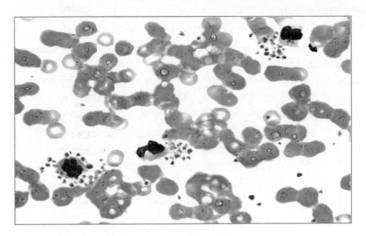

a. Describe platelet satellitism.
b. What is its clinical significance?
c. How do you take care of such a situation?

Q46. Answer the following questions.

a. What is the effect on PT and PTT in hemophilia A?
b. Calculate the dose of factor VIII required, to increase factor VIII levels by 50%, in a child weighing 10 kg
c. Give the other name for hemophilia C.
d. Give 2 examples of gene therapy being tried for hemophilia.

Q47. A 5-year-old child presented with pallor and cutaneous markers at the back with an abnormal skeletal profile. Peripheral smear was consistent with macrocytic anemia and pancytopenia.

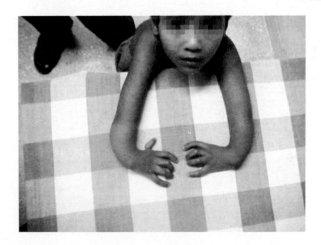

a. What is the most probable diagnosis?
b. Name the cutaneous marker.
c. What malignancies are expected in this patient?

Q48. A previously asymptomatic 5-year-old girl is referred with an abdominal mass found by her mother as she was undressing her. On examination, a mass arising from right renal angle is noted which extends medially almost up to midline and inferiorly 10 cm. Her BP is 160/110 mm Hg. Investigations show normal plasma urea, creatinine and electrolytes. Urine examination reveals hematuria but culture is sterile.

a. Give the 2 most likely differential diagnoses?
b. What is the mechanism of raised blood pressure?
c. For each diagnosis give one site where metastases might be commonly found.

ANSWERS

A 1:

a. Fresh Frozen Plasma
b. 300 mL (15 mL/kg)
c.
    i. Severe clotting factor deficiency and bleeding
    ii. Severe clotting factor deficiency and invasive procedure
    iii. Emergency reversal of warfarin effects
    iv. Dilutional coagulopathy and bleeding.

A 2:

a. Idiopathic pulmonary hemosiderosis
b. BAL showing hemosiderin laden macrophages or gastric lavage showing siderophages or lung biopsy
c. Steroids.

A 3:

a. Diagnosis: Hodgkin disease
b. Classification: WHO classification
    Classical HL
    – Nodular sclerosis
    – mixed cellularity
    – lymphocyte depleted
    – lymphocyte-rich classical HL
    Nodular lymphocyte predominant HL
c. Staging: Ann Arbor Staging
d. Drugs: Adriamycin, bleomycin, vinblastin, dacarbazine.

A 4:

a. Familial HLH (Hemophagocytic lymphohistiocytosis)
b. High ferritin, high triglyceride
c. EBV, CMV, HIV, HSV, HHV 6–8, rubella, varicella, parvo, TB, Brucella, Mycoplasma, leishmania.

A 5:

a. APTT
b. RICE: Rest, Ice, compression, elevation
c. If hemophila A: Factor 8
    If hemophilia B: Factor 9.

A 6:

a. Wiskott Aldrich syndrome
b. Small platelets (Low MPV < 7), Immunoglobulin levels: Low IgM
c. Hematopoeietic stem cell transplant
d. Untreated disease is fatal secondary to infections or bleeding. Long term risks of leukemia and lymphomas.

A 7:

a. Burkitts lymphoma or B cell NHL
b. Double maintenance fluids and allopurinol
c. Rasburicase
d. Starry sky appearance
e. 70–80% overall survival.

A 8:

a. Diagnosis: Aplastic anemia
b. Two important investigations can be
   - Chromosomal breakage study
   - PNH study
c. Hep B, C, HIV, Hep A, EBV, CMV
   - Options of treatment
   - Bone marrow transplant
   - Immunosuppressive therapy with ATG and cyclosporin.

A 9:

a. Reticulocyte
b. Supravital stain (new methylene blue or brilliant cresyl blue).
c. 0.5–2%
d. Elevated in:
   - Hemolytic anemias like AIHA, HS
   - Blood loss.

A 10:

a. Dyskeratosis congenita
b. Short telomere length
c. BMT or androgens
d. Malignancies like leukemias or head and neck cancers.

A 11:

a. Acute leukemia most likely ALL
b. Flowcytometry
c. Vincristine, steroids, daunorubicin, L asparaginase, methotrexate, cyclophosphamide, cytarabine, 6 MP
d. 70–80% cure rate of 5 year survival.

A 12:

a. Hypersegmented neutrophil
b. Megaloblastic anemia
c. Parenteral B_{12} or oral folic acid therapy.

A 13:

a. HIV associated immune thrombocytopenia
b. HIV ELISA
c. Antiretroviral drugs. Chronic ITP may need IVIg, anti D, steroids, dapsone, eltrombopag

A 14:

a. Thalassemia minor
b. HPLC, HbA2 >3.4%, rest normal
c. No therapy.

A 15:

a. Neuroblastoma stage IV
b. Urinary catecholamines
c. Biopsy from the abdominal mass
d. Adrenal grand or the parasympathetic ganglia.

A 16:

a. Neuroblastoma with opsoclonus myoclonus
b. Surgical removal of the mass, steroids, IVIG
c. Excellent outcome

A 17:

a. T lymphoblastic lymphoma
b. Cytopathology and Flowcytometry of the pleural fluid
c. Never attempt a mediastinal biopsy, avoid sedation and intubation
d. Keep the patient in propped up position. Start steroids empirically.

A 18:

a. Acute leukemia with tumor lysis syndrome
b. Hyperkalemia, hyperuricemia, hypocalcemia, hyperphosphatemia, deranged renal functions
c. Double maintenance Fluids, allopurinol, phosphate binders in case of high phosphorus, avoid IV calcium.

A 19:

a. Hb H/Hb CS disease with hemolytic crisis
b. Preceding viral infections.

A 20:

a. Selective IgA deficiency
b. Avoid blood products and immunoglobulin preparations (use product that has been depleted of IgA).

A 21:

a. Pseudohypoxemia due to oxygen consumption by high TLC.
b. Analyze sample immediately after drawing or send the sample on ice.

A 22:

a. Iron deficiency anemia.
b. Iron at 4–6 mg/kg/day (elemental).
c. Subjective improvement, decreased irritability and increased apetite within 12–24 hours.

A 23:
a. Methemoglobin level $\geq$15%.
b. 85%.
c. Injection methylene blue 1–2 mg/kg IV. Daily vitamin C 200–500 mg in divided doses also used (but not for toxic methemoglobinemia).
d. G6PD deficiency.
e. Oxygen saturation will be low but the arterial blood gas will show a normal or high PaO_2 (if receiving oxygen therapy).

A 24:
a. Histiocytosis.
b. Lytic lesions in bone.
c. Histiocytes.
d. Birbeck granules on electron microscopy.

A 25:
a. Target cell.
b. • Thalassemia.
   • Hemoglobinopathies—Hb AC or CC, Hb SS, SC, S-thal.
   • Liver disease.
   • Postsplenectomy or hyposplenic states.
   • Severe iron deficiency.
   • HbE (hetro and homozygous).
   • LCAT deficiency.
   • Abetalipoprotenemia.

A 26:
a. ANA, ds DNA, HIV, serum immunoglobulin.
b. • Platelet transfusion.
   • Methyl prednisolone—500 mg/m² IV /day × 3 days.
   • IV IG 0.8–1.0 g/kg.
   • Anti-D therapy for Rh positive patients.
   • Emergency splenectomy.
c. Indications for bone marrow aspirations include an abnormal WBC count or differential or unexplained anemia as well as finding suggestive of bone marrow disease on history and physical examination.
d. When thrombocytopenia persists for more than 6 months.
e. Valproic acid, phenytoin, sulfonamides, cotrimoxazole.

A 27:
a. Hemophilia A or B.
b. PTT increased.
c. X-linked recessive.
d. Moderate:
   • Severe: <1% activity of specific clotting factor and spontaneous bleeding
   • Moderate: 1–5%; require mild trauma to induce bleeding
   • Mild: >5%; require significant trauma to cause bleeding.

A 28:

a. Sickle cell beta + thalassemia.
b. Beta + thalassemia.
c. *Streptococcus pneumoniae, Haemophilus influenzae* type B.

A 29:

a. Kawasaki disease
b. Alpha thalassemia major
c. Beta thalassemia major
d. Sickle cell disease
e. G6PD deficiency
f. Hereditary spherocytosis

1. Thrombocytosis
2. Hydrops fetalis
3. Increased fetal Hb
4. Hyposplenism in a 6-year-old
5. Oxidant induced red cell damage
6. Splenomegaly in a 6-year-old

A 30:

a. Acute lymphoblastic leukemia.
b. 2–6 years; more common in boys than girls at all ages.
c. ALL is diagnosed by a bone marrow evaluation that demonstrates >25% of the bone marrow cells as a homogeneous population of lymphoblasts.
d. • Age <1 year or >10 years at diagnosis
   • Leukocyte count of >100,000/mm^3 at diagnosis
   • Slow response to initial therapy
   • Chromosomal abnormalities, including hypodiploidy, the philadelphia chromosome, and MLL gene rearrangements and translocations [t(1:19) or t(4;11)]
   • CNS involvement at presentation.

A 31:

a. This represents an example of iron-deficiency anemia. The history should include details of birth (prematurity, excessive blood loss from placenta) and diet (amount of milk intake, food containing iron).
b. Limit the amount of milk in the diet and increase the amount of iron containing food (cereals).
c. To continue iron supplementation for six months. Repeat Hb levels after a month.

A 32:

a. Microcytic Hypochromic anemia with few target cells and tear drop cells. WBC and platelets appear normal.
b. Iron deficiency anemia; thalassemia; sideroblastic anemia, lead poisoning.
c. • Serum iron/TIBC
   • Hemoglobin electrophoresis
   • Bone marrow study.

A 33:

a. • Langerhans cell histiocytosis
   • Familial erythrophagocytic lymphohistiocytosis
   • Infection associated hemophagocytic syndrome.

b i. • Malignant histiocytosis
    • Acute monocytic leukemia
    • Seborrheic dermatitis/petechia:
  ii. Hypothalamic involvement/pituitary dysfunction—diabetes insipidus/primary hypothyroidism.
  iii. Osteolytic lesion in bones with no evidence of reactive new bone formation/fractures/vertebral collapse/floating teeth.
c. Hyperlipidemia, hypofibrinogenimia, elevated liver enzymes, extremely elevated circulating interlukin 2 receptors.

A 34:

a. Acute leukemia.
b. Bone marrow aspirate and biopsy.
c. ALL and AML.
d. No.
e. Yes; chloroma.

Characteristic	Myeloblast	Lymphoblast
Size	Larger	Smaller
Cytoplasm	Moderate	Scanty
Auer rods	May be present	Absent
Nuclear chromatin	Fine	Coarse
Nucleoli	Prominent, 1-4	Indistinct

A 35:

a. Macrocytic anemia.
b. • Folic acid deficiency (nutritional).
    • Vitamin B_{12} deficiency (nutritional).
    • Pernicious anemia.
    • Malabsorption disorders.
    • Surgical resection of bowel.
c. Anticonvulsants—phenytoin, phenobarbitone
   Antifolate–methorexate, pryrimethamine.

A 36:

a. Microcytic hypochromic anemia.
b. Iron-deficiency anemia, thalassemia, lead poisoning, sideroblastic anemia.
c. RDW is red cell distribution width and RDW is increased in iron-deficiency anemia.

A 37:

a. Sickle cell anemia.

b. Hemoglobin S (Hb S) is the result of a single base pair change, thymine for adenine, at the 6th codon of the β-globin gene. This change encodes valine instead of glutamine in the 6th position in the β-globin molecule.

c. Human parvovirus B19.

A 38:

a. Blasts seen—most likely lymphoblasts.

b. ALL.

c. Down syndrome, Bloom syndrome, ataxia-telangiectasia, and Fanconi's syndrome.

d. Epstein-Barr viral infections.

A 39:

a. Band cell—Immature neutrophil.

b. 6 hours.

c. Phenothiazines, sulfonamides, anticonvulsants, penicillins, aminopyrine.

A 40:

a. Severe combined immunodeficiency (SCID).

b. Bone marrow transplant before 3½ months of life.

c. Give irradiated blood products to prevent GVHD.

A 41:

a. Leukocyte adhesion deficiency.

b. *Staphylococcus aureus, E.coli , Candida* and *Aspergillus.*

c. Early allogenic bone marrow transplantation.

A 42:

Disease	Deficiencies
a. Lupus-like syndrome	C1 Q
b. Recurrent neisserial infections	C5, 6, 7, 8, 9 C3
c. Severe recurrent pneumococcal infection	C3
d. Fatal meningococcal infections in males	Properdin
e. Nonpitting edema	C1 inhibitor

A 43:

a. Pentad:
   i. Thrombocytopenia
   ii. Microangiopathic hemolytic anemia
   iii. Neurological abnormalities
   iv. Renal dysfunction
   v. Fever.

b. Congenital deficiency of metalloproteinase can result in familial TTP.

c. Plasmapheresis. (Corticosteroids and splenectomy reserved for refractory cases).

d. Morphologically abnormal RBC with schistocytes, spherocytes, helmet cells and increased reticulocyte count in association with thrombocytopenia.

A 44:

a. Two macrophages are shown which have a fibrillar, crumpled appearing cytoplasm and eccentric nuclei, consistent with Gaucher cells. The other hematopoietic elements present are normal.
b. Niemann Pick disease, MPS, granulocytic leukemia and myeloma.
c. Enzyme replacement (acid beta glucosidase) 60 units/kg, IV on alternate week and then monthly maintenance, bone marrow transplant.

A 45:

a. Platelet satellitism: Platelet clustering around neutrophils in the presence of EDTA.
b. Pseudothrombocytopenia.
c. Repeat platelet count in citrate sample.

A 46:

a. PT–normal ; PTT–increased.
b. 250 units.
c. von Willibrand disease.
d. Adeno associated virus (AAV), plasmid infection in fibroblasts, retroviruses.

A 47:

a. Fanconi anemia.
b. Café au lait spot.
c. Acute leukemia.

A 48:

a. Wilm's tumour and neuroblastoma.
b. • Wilm's tumour—renal ischemia.
   • Neuroblastoma—increased catecholamines secretion.
c. • Wilm's tumour—lungs.
   • Neuroblastoma—long bones.

QUESTIONS

Q1. A 4-year-old female presents with ulcers on her tongue and oral mucosa. The patient refuses to eat due to pain in her mouth. Her temperature is 102 F. A rash is noted on hands, feet and buttocks.

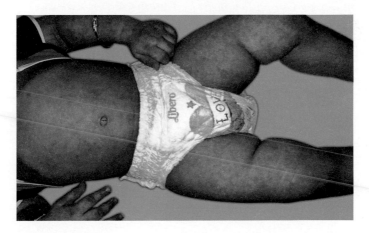

a. What is the diagnosis?
b. What is the causative organism?
c. How is it transmitted?
d. What is the treatment?

Q2. An infant girl is born 4 weeks prematurely and manifests jaundice, an intractable rash, persistent rhinitis, pneumonia, anemia, generalized lymphadenopathy, and bony abnormalities on radiograph.

a. What is the most likely diagnosis?
b. What historical features is the most important when questioning the mother regarding the history of the pregnancy?
c. What findings would most likely be present on ophthalmic examination of this newborn child?
d. What is the famous triad and its association in older children?

Q3. Select the answers

a. Neonatal herpes
b. Congenital cytomegalovirus infection
c. Congenital toxoplasmosis
d. Congenital syphilis
e. Congenital varicella
    i. Sensorineural deafness
    ii. Limb abnormalities
    iii. Short stature
    iv. Glaucoma
    v. Hydrocephalus
    vi Tram-track calcifications
    vii. Saddle nose
    viii. Skin, eye, mouth infections.

Q4. Pulmonary Koch's

a. Write drug therapy of a 10 kg boy according to IAP guideline.

Q5. Pulmonary Koch's, Complete the table below

Treatment Categories and Regimens for Childhood Tuberculosis

Category of treatment	Type of patients	TB treatment regimens	
		Intensive phase	*Continuation Phase*
New cases	• New smear-positive pulmonary Tuberculosis (PTB) • New smear-negative PTB • New extra-pulmonary TB	A	B
Previously treated cases	• Relapse, failure to respond or treatment after default • Re-treatment Others	C	D

Q6. RMNCH+A

a. What is RMNCH+A?
b. When was it launched?
c. Targets- Fill in the xblanks
    i. Reduction of infant mortality rate (IMR) to_____per 1,000 live births by 2017
    ii. Reduction in maternal mortality ratio (MMR) to_____per 100,000 live births by 2017
    iii. Reduction in total fertility rate (TFR) to_____by 2017.

Q7. A 12 year 32 kg presents with active pulmonary tuberculosis. He previously has taken treatment for 6 weeks and comes after interruption of treatment for 1 year.

a. What category of treatment shall this child fall in?

b. Which patients are candidate for *Extending intensive and continuation phase*?
c. *What is the guideline for TB preventive therapy*

Q 8.

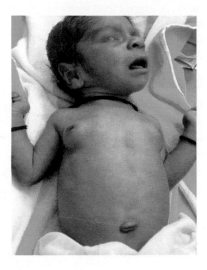

a. What is the diagnosis?
b. What is the most common organism associated with the said abnormality?
c. What is the treatment?

Q9. This 4 years old child has the lesions shown below which are itching in nature. Lesions were also there in the groins, male genitalia and between the buttocks.

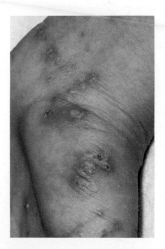

a. What is the likely diagnosis?
b. What is the organism causing above problems?
c. What is the treatment?

Q10. Answer the following questions on malaria.

a. Define drug sensitive malaria.
b. What are the grades of resistance?
c. What are the indications for use of primaquine in the treatment of malaria?

Q11. A 15-year-old female presents with fever for past 24 hours. Fever is high grade associated with sweating and loose motions (10 large, watery stools over past 6 hours). For past 2 hours patient is complaining of giddiness. 5 days back (prior to fever) patient had her menses which were of normal duration and normal blood loss. On examination—Toxic looking, drowsy with Glasgow coma scale of 10. Blood pressure systolic 70 mm Hg, pulse rate 140/min, capillary fill time 4 seconds, RR–30/min. There is diffuse erythematous macular rash (sun burn like) all over body.

a. What is the most probable diagnosis?
b. What is the first step in management other than airway and breathing?
c. What class (targeting particular bacteria) of antibiotic you would like to give to this patient?
d. Name common predisposing factor which can cause above mentioned disease.
e. Intravenous immunoglobulin has no role to play in the above mentioned disease at any level: (Write true/false).

Q12. Study this picture of a 8-month-old infant who developed a rash during the declining phase of fever starting with the cheeks.

a. What is the most probable diagnosis?
b. What is the causative organism?
c. Name two situations where infection with this organism may be life threatening.

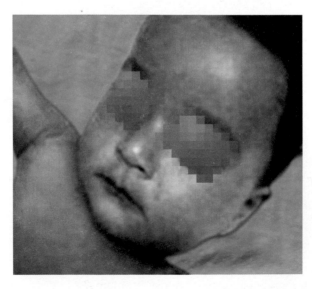

Q13. A one-year-old child presented with fever, barking cough and breathing difficulties. Initially child was having only running nose. O/E: Tachypnea, stridor, subcostal retractions and intercostal retractions.

a. What is the diagnosis?
b. What is the usual etiological agent?
c. Which X-ray sign is diagnostic of this condition?

Q14. This 8-day-old female baby (shown in photograph) was brought to PHC with complaints of progressive difficulty in feeding, crying excessively and seizures. Parents of baby were 2nd degree cousins and laborers by occupation. Mother had not received any antenatal care. Baby was born at home, had moderate cry, and was well till day-8. On examination: HR–140/min; RR–42/min; AF–at level; sutures–normal. Tone–Increased in all 4 limbs with neck retraction, intermittent seizures, worsening with stimulus.

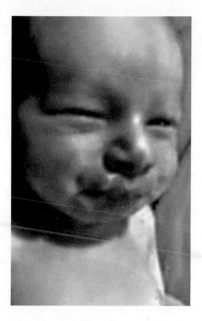

a. What is the diagnosis of this baby?
b. What is the treatment?
c. What is the usual cause of death in this condition?
d. What are the various types of this disease?
e. Excision of umbilical stump is recommended in this case (state true/false).

Q15. During a prenatal visit, an HIV seropositive woman asks you about the advisability of breast-feeding.

a. How would you counsel her if she is from educated, well to do family from an urban area like Delhi?
b. If she is uneducated and poor from rural India?
c. How your advice would differ, if at all, she was HbsAg +ve positive instead?

Q16. A 7-year-old male presents with headache, fever and vomiting for past 24 hours. Fever is high grade associated with sweating. For past 2 hours patient is complaining of uneasiness, headache and vomiting. On examination–Toxic looking, drowsy with Glasgow coma scale of 8. Blood pressure systolic–50 mm Hg, pulse rate 140/min, capillary fill time 4 seconds, RR–30/min. There is rash (petechial) over abdomen and limbs.

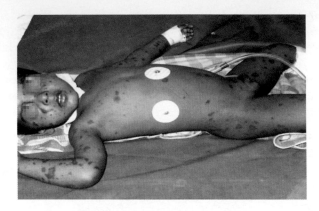

a. What is the most probable diagnosis?
b. What is the first step in management other than airway and breathing?
c. What class (targeting particular bacteria) of antibiotic you would like to give to this patient?
d. What drug you would like to give in dopamine refractory shock?

Q17. When the mother is HIV positive:

a. What is the percentage of transmission of HIV through breast milk?
b. What should the mother be appraised of, if she chooses to breast feed her baby?
c. What are the methods by which breast milk can be processed to reduce chances of transmission?
d. What criteria should be taken into account if mother wants to feed the baby with formula milk?

Q18. Study the two pictures shown below and answer the following questions.

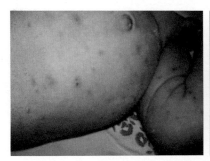
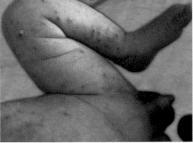

a. Outline the treatment for this condition.
b. List 4 complications of this condition.
c. Any medications you would advise for his 5 years old elder sister and his mother who is 2 months pregnant?

Q19. A primigravida mother who had a history of fever with vesiculo-pustular rash during second trimester of pregnancy gives birth to a IUGR baby having cicatricial skin lesions and hypoplasia of certain fingers and toes. Neuroimaging of this baby revealed cortical atrophy with ventriculomegaly.
a. What is the diagnosis?
b. List 3 clinical features of this condition.
c. What percentage of fetus may get infected if a pregnant lady gets this infection in early pregnancy?

Q20. A 3-year-old female child is a newly diagnosed case of HIV. Write down the prescription (names only) for this patient with protease inhibitor based regimens keeping in mind her latest investigations, which are; CD4 cell count is 70/mm³ and the percentage of this is <15% of total lymphocytes. Her Hb is 9.2 g%, platelets are 1.6 lacs/mm³ and normal LFT.

Q21. A 5-year-old child has sustained a bleeding injury on left leg due to exposure to the paws of a clinically rabid dog. There was definitely no bite or saliva contamination of the wound.
a. What class of bite (injury) is this?
b. How would you manage this patient?

Q 22. A 5-year-old male child is brought to ER with fever, edema of left eyelid, redness and proptosis. There is severe pain on touching the area. There is a history of penetrating lid trauma 6 hours back while playing. The child is also diabetic and on regular insulin therapy.
a. What is the diagnosis?
b. Mention two most likely causative organisms.
c. Mention three complications of this entity.

Q 23. A 3-year-old boy presented with failure to thrive. The child was apparently asymptomatic for the first two years of life. He began to have diarrhea with light colored stools. Although stool examinations were performed, it was unclear what the report is. The child was placed on a high protein, high calorie diet with vitamins and supplements. However, he showed very little improvement over a 4 month period. Barium exam showed "large dilated loops of hypotonic bowel", the child was admitted with a suspicion of celiac disease. Stool examination shows a flagellated protozoan parasite, which on staining shows a characteristic "smiley face" symbols.
a. Identify the condition.
b. What is the best possible diagnostic test?
c. How do you treat this condition?

Q24. A 8-year-old child resident of Delhi is admitted with fever for last 5-6 days, loss of appetite for 6 days and hepatosplenomegaly. His peripheral smear is shown below.

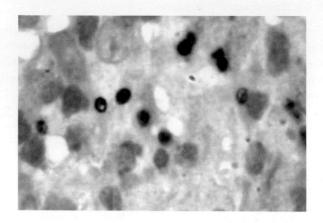

a. Identify the picture (name the form of parasite).
b. Name the culture media used for growth of this parasite.
c. Name the drugs used to treat resistant cases infected with this parasite.

Q25. A pregnant lady found to be HBsAg positive, gives birth to a term baby.

a. What is the risk of the baby getting hepatitis B infection?
b. How do you protect the baby?
c. Is there a possibility for the baby to be infected in spite of proper management?
d. What is the prognosis in the infected newborns?

Q26. A 7-year-old boy presented with 4 weeks history of high grade fever, fatigue, weight loss and was found to have a grossly enlarged relatively non tender liver 4 cm below costal margin and spleen 6 cm but no lymphadenopathy. His Hb was 4 g%, TLC was 3500 cells/mm³ and platelet counts of 56,000 mm³. A bone marrow aspiration was done and the slide is depicted below.

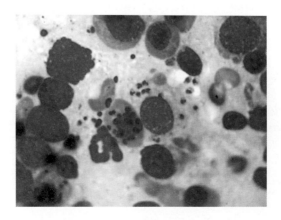

a. Describe the findings on smear and give the diagnosis.
b. Name the first line drug for the condition. Write the dose, route of administration and duration.
c. Name two other drugs for this condition.

Q27. A 7-year-old boy, resident of UP comes home from school daily by walking through a paddy field. Near his home are found many stray cattle and other wild animals like pigs. Two days ago he developed high grade fever, headache and vomiting. Ten hours later he developed multiple seizures and became unconscious. On examination, there is no pallor, he is febrile, comatose and has generalized hypertonia and a left hemiparesis. There are no signs of meningeal irritation. There is no hepatosplenomegaly. He has received all childhood immunizations appropriate for his age. There is history of similar cases in the area in the preceding two weeks.

a. What is the likely clinical diagnosis?
b. How is this disease transmitted?
c. What are the methods to confirm the diagnosis?
d. What is the test of choice?

Q28. A 5-year-old male child presents with fever for past 10 days. Fever is high grade, continuous in nature without chills and rigor. There are no associated loose motions, vomiting, headache, photophobia, cough, cold or rash. On examination child is conscious, febrile, normotensive with conjunctival congestion but no discharge. Two cervical lymph nodes (Right sided) are palpable, approximately 2 cm each. There is desquamation of the skin around the fingers. There is no hepatosplenomegaly. Rest of systemic examination is normal.

a. What is your most probable diagnosis?
b. Name one characteristic feature that can be found in complete blood counts.
c. In what percentage of cases does the acute illness tend to recur?
d. What drug (drug of choice) you would like to give to this patient?

Q29. A 14-year-old female child complains of pain in abdomen for past 10 days. She has also developed vomiting and loose motions for past 4 days. She also has weakness of both lower limbs and is unable to walk past 24 hours. On examination—she is hypertensive, with a HR 142/min. CNS examination reveals diminished tone in both her lower limbs with power grade 2. Deep tendon reflexes are not elicitable.

a. Give 2 differential diagnoses for this condition.
b. Investigations revealed serum Na^+–110 mEq/L, K^+–4 mEq/L, SGPT–37 U/L.
   She is passing high colored urine —What is the probable diagnosis?
c. Suggest one investigation for diagnosis.
d. Suggest the appropriate treatment.

Q30. A male child aged 13-month-old presented with loose motions for 5 days. On 2nd day of loose motions, he passed blood along with stools. On the 4th day of illness loose motions stopped but he also developed decreased urine output. He became irritable, and had one episode of abnormal movements with altered sensorium 1 hour back. Parents were giving ORS for past 3 days. Weaning was started 3 months back. On examination—the child is pale, and also has petechiae, hepatomegaly, tachypnea and edema. His BP is 100/60 mm Hg. There is mild acidosis on ABG.

a. Name two differential diagnoses.
b. Name 3 electrolyte disturbances that can be associated with the illness.
c. What would be your management plan?

Q31. A 12-year-old male presented with pain in abdomen for past 8 days (acute intermittent, periumbilical). He also developed swelling over the scrotum 6 days back which subsided within 24 hours. During the past 2 days, he has developed pain over right wrist and swelling of the right knee. He also developed rash over both lower legs and gluteal region. This morning his stools were bright red. Abdominal palpation reveals generalized tenderness and the right lower quadrant is empty.

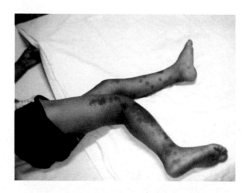

a. What is your most probable diagnoses?

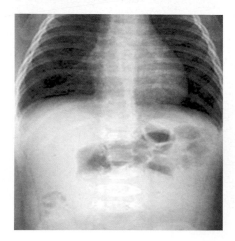

b. X-ray abdomen is shown above—What complication has the patient developed?

c. What is the definitive medical treatment (specific for disease—other than blood/resuscitative fluid)?

Q32. A 4-year-old female child presented with gradually increasing difficulty in breathing with cough and fever for past 10 hours. She had one episode of hemoptysis and 1-2 episodes of malena 24 hours back. On examination, she is pale, HR–162/min and RR–50/min. Examination of respiratory system shows bilateral wheezing. Blood investigations showed microcytic hypochromic anemia with reticulocytosis. Serum iron was found to be low.

a. What is the diagnosis?

b. What is the diagnostic investigation with findings?

c. Which cardiac condition can resemble such symptomatology?

Q33. Match the appropriate antidote to its corresponding drug overdose.

a.	Desferoxamine	1. Acetaminophen
b.	N-Acetyl cysteine	2. Benzodiazepine
c.	Pyridoxine	3. Nitrates/methemoglobinemia
d.	Vitamin K	4. Isoniazid
e.	BAL	5. Heavy metals (mercury, gold, arsenic)
f.	Methylene blue	6. Organophosphate
g.	Atropine	7. Iron
h.	Flumazenil	8. Coumarin

Q34. Study the given CT scan of head.

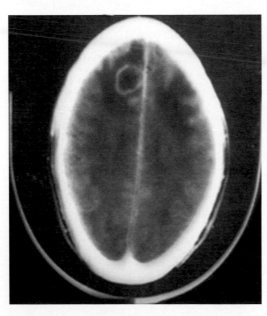

Answer questions based on CT head shown above

a. What does this CT scan head reveal?
b. What is the likely diagnosis?
c. Name the drugs used in medical management of this condition.
d. What are the indications for surgical interventions in such a case?

Q35. Answer the questions based on the picture shown below. This child was systemically unwell with fever.

a. What is the diagnosis?
b. Name two causes for this condition.
c. What sites are commonly affected in this condition?

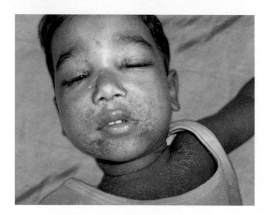

Q36. A 5-year-old male child residing in an overcrowded slum, presents with itchy lesions in the groins, male genitalia and between the buttocks.

a. Spot the diagnosis and name the etiological agent.
b. What is the treatment for this condition?

Q37. A 7-year-old male child presented with sudden onset explosive watery diarrhea with abdominal distension, flatulence and epigastric cramps without any blood or mucus in the stool. Stool examination of this child is shown below.

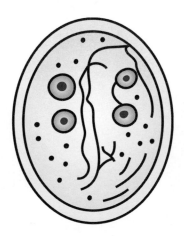

a. What is the diagnosis?
b. What would be the schedule for stool microscopic examination for this condition?
c. Name two other modalities of diagnosis other than stool microscopy.
d. What are the drugs used in treatment? (At least 3).

Q38. A 18-year-old student presents to OPD with 10 days history of fever, sore throat, malaise, and a rash that developed today. Fever was initially low grade but rose to 103°F (39.4°C) 4 days ago. She has worsening sore throat and difficulty swallowing solid foods but she is drinking well. She denies emesis, diarrhea, or sick contacts.

On examination, there is a diffuse morbilliform rash over the body. She appears tired but in no distress. Her temperature is 102.2°F (39°C). She has mild supraorbital edema, bilaterally enlarged tonsils that are coated with a shaggy gray exudate; a few petechiae on the palate and uvula; bilateral posterior cervical lymphadenopathy; and a spleen that is palpable 3 cm below the costal margin. Laboratory data include a white blood cell (WBC) count of 17,000 cells/mm³ with 50% lymphocytes, 15% atypical lymphocytes, and platelet count of 100,000/mm³.

a. What is the most likely diagnosis?
b. What is the best tool to quickly confirm this diagnosis?
c. What is the best management for this condition?
d. What is the expected course of this condition?

ANSWERS

A 1:

a. Hand foot and mouth disease.
b. Entero virus group including polio viruses, coxsackie viruses, echo viruses, and entero viruses. Coxsackie A virus is the commonest virus causing HFMD.
c. An infected person may spread the viruses that cause hand, foot, and mouth disease to another person through:
  - Close personal contact
  - Air droplets (through coughing or sneezing)
  - Contact with feces
  - Contact with contaminated objects and surfaces.
d. Supportive, adequate liquid intake and pain relief

A 2:

a. Congenital syphilis
b. Sexual history
c. Segmental pigmentation of the retinal periphery, salt and pepper appearance to the fundus
d. Hutchinson's triad—interstitial Keratitis, widely spaced and peg-shaped teeth, Deafness

A 3:

a. 8
b. 1
c. 5
d. 7
e. 2

A 4:

- Intensive phase 2 months
- 3 days a week
- Isoniazid 100 mg
- Rifampicin 100–120 mg
- Pyrazinamide 300–350 mg
- Ethambutol 200–250 mg
- Continuation phase 4 months
- 3 days a week
- Isoniazid 100 mg
- Rifampicin 100–120 mg.

The following are the daily doses (mg per kg of body weight per day)
- Rifampicin 10–12 mg/kg (max 600 mg/day)
- Isoniazid 10 mg/kg (max 300 mg/day)
- Ethambutol 20–25 mg/kg (max 1500 mg/day)
- PZA 30-35 mg/kg (max 2000 mg/day) and
- Streptomycin 15 mg/kg (max 1g/day).

A 5:

a. $2H_3R_3Z_3E_3$
b. $4H_3R_3$
c. $2S_3H_3R_3Z_3E_3 + 1H_3R_3Z_3E_3$
d. $5H_3R_3E_3$

Category of treatment	Type of patients	TB treatment regimens	
		Intensive phase	Continuation phase
New cases	• New smear-positive pulmonary Tuberculosis (PTB) • New smear-negative PTB • New extra-pulmonary TB	$2H_3R_3Z_3E_3$*	$4H_3R_3$
Previously treated cases	• Relapse, failure to respond or treatment after default • Re-treatment Others	$2S_3H_3R_3Z_3E_3$ $+1H_3R_3Z_3E_3$	$5H_3R_3E_3$

H=Isoniazid, R= Rifampicin, Z= Pyrazinamide, E= Ethambutol, S= Streptomycin. *The number before the letters refers to the number of months of treatment. The subscript after the letters refers to the number of doses per week. Pulmonary TB refers to disease involving lung parenchyma.

A 6:

a. Reproductive, maternal, newborn, child and adolescent health
b. 2013
c. Targets
    i. Reduction of infant mortality rate (IMR) to 25 per 1,000 live births by 2017
    ii. Reduction in maternal mortality ratio (MMR) to 100 per 100,000 live births by 2017
    iii. Reduction in Total Fertility Rate (TFR) to 2.1 by 2017

A 7:

i. Default
    ii. a. Children who show inadequate or no response (on smear or clinico-radiological basis) at 8 weeks of intensive phase should be given benefit of extension of IP for one more month.
        b. In patients with TB meningitis, spinal TB, miliary/disseminated TB and osteo-articular TB, the continuation phase shall be extended by 3 months making the total duration of treatment to a total of 9 months. A further extension may be done for 3 more months in continuation phase (making the total duration of treatment to 12 months) on a case to case basis in case of delayed response and as per the discretion of the treating physician/ pediatrician.
    iii. a. All asymptomatic contacts (under 6 years of age) of a smear positive case, after ruling out active disease and irrespective of their BCG, TST or nutritional status.

b. Chemoprophylaxis is also recommended for all HIV infected children who either had a known exposure to an infectious TB case or are tuberculin skin test (TST) positive (≥5 mm induration) but have no active TB disease.

c. All TST positive children who are receiving immunosuppressive therapy (e.g. Children with nephrotic syndrome, acute leukemia, etc.).

d. A child born to mother who was diagnosed to have TB in pregnancy should receive prophylaxis for 6 months, provided congenital TB has been ruled out. BCG vaccination can be given at birth even if INH chemoprophylaxis is planned.

A 8:

a. Mastitis neonatorum—Secreting tissue in neonatal breasts
b. *Staphylococcus aureus*
c. Antimicronbial therapy
   Needle aspiration/Incision and drainage in rare case.

A 9:

a. Scabies
b. Sarcoptes scabei (Mite)
c. 5% permethrin cream for local application x 10 hrs
   All family members to be treated simultaneously
   All linen and cloths to be cleaned (boil put out in the sun and subject to hot iron)
   Treatment may be repeated 2 weeks later
   (Oral ivermectin after 5 years of age)

A 10:

a. Sensitive to drugs if clearance of asexual parasitemia by day 6 from initiation of treatment without subsequent recrudescence until day 28.

b. Resistance to drugs: R1, R2, R3.
   R1—Clearance of asexual parasitemia for at least 2 consecutive days, latest by day 6, after initiation of treatment, followed by recrudescence within day 28.
   R2—Marked reduction of asexual parasitemia to less than 25% of pretreatment counts within 48 hours of initiation of treatment, but with no subsequent disappearance of asexual parasitemia (positive on day 6 after initiation of treatment).
   R3—Modest reduction (not < 25%), no change or increase in asexual parasitemia during first 48 hours following implementation of treatment and no subsequent clearance of asexual parasitemia.

c. Primaquine is used as a gametocidal agent for *P. falciparum*—0.75 mg/kg single dose and in *P. vivax* to prevent recrudescence at a dose of 0.25 mg/kg/day for 5 days.

A 11:

a. Toxic shock syndrome.
b. Management of shock, fluid boluses.
c. Anti-staphylococcal drugs.
d. Use of tampoons or vaginal device.
e. False.

A 12:

a. Erythema infectiosum/fifth disease.
b. Parvovirus B_{19}.
c. Life threatening situations:
   - Aplastic crisis in hemolytic anemia
   - Non-immune hydrops fetalis in fetal infection.

A 13:

a. Croup.
b. Para influenza A.
c. Steeple sign (on lateral X-ray neck).

A 14:

a. Neonatal tetanus.
b. • Penicillin G-1 lakh units/kg/day q 4-6 hourly IV for 10-14 days
   • Tetanus immunoglobulin, muscle relaxants—Diazepam, baclofen
   • $MgSO_4$, midazolam
   • NM blockers—Pancuronium, vecuronium.
c. Recurrent spasms causing airway obstruction.
d. Neonatal, localized, generalized, cephalic.
e. False.

A 15:

a. In Delhi she should refrain from breast-feeding, where safe alternatives to breast-feeding are available. Both free and cell-associated viruses have been detected in breast milk from HIV-infected mothers. The additional risk for transmission through breast-feeding in women with HIV infection before pregnancy is 14% compared with a 29% increase in breast-feeding women who acquired HIV postnatally. This suggests that the viremia experienced by the mother during primary infection doubles the risk for transmission. It therefore seems reasonable for women to substitute infant formula for breast milk if they are known to be HIV-infected.

b. In rural India, because of infectious disease and malnutrition, breast-feeding would be continued. WHO recommends that in developing countries where other diseases (diarrhea, pneumonia, malnutrition) substantially contribute to a high infant mortality rate, the benefit of breast-feeding outweighs the risk for HIV transmission, and HIV-infected women in developing countries should breast-feed their infants for the 1st 6 months of life followed by rapid weaning.

c. If HBsAg is positive, infant should receive hepatitis B immunoglobulin and hepatitis B vaccine within 24 hours of birth (no later than 72 hours) and hepatitis B vaccine at 6 and 14 weeks or 6 weeks and 6 months and breastfeeding should be given.

A 16:

a. Meningococcemia.
b. Management of shock, fluid boluses.
c. Ceftriaxone.
d. Steroids.

A 17:

a. • 14% if mother acquired infection before pregnancy.
   • 29% increased risk if mother acquired infection during pregnancy.
b. i. Benefits of breastfeeding.
   ii. Risk of transmission while breastfeeding (e.g. through cracked nipple).
   iii. To avoid mixed feeding and to rapidly wean off breastfeeds by the end of 6th month of life.
   iv. Mother should be on ART while feeding.
c. i. Pasteurized breast milk.
   ii. Boiled human milk.
   iii. Frozen human milk.
   iv. Expressed breast milk allowed to stand and remove the lipid layer.
d. • Acceptability.
   • Affordability.
   • Sustainability.
   • Safety and feasibility.

A 18: Varicella

a. Symptomatic treatment with antipyretics/antihistamines/hygiene, etc. is advised if child is healthy and is suffering from uncomplicated varicella. Acyclovir is started within 72 hours if child is immunosuppressed/on steroids or on salicylates/has chronic cardiac or pulmonary disorder or is having complicated varicella.
b. • Secondary bacterial skin infections.
   • Encephalitis/cerebellar ataxia.
   • Pneumonia.
   • Purpura/HUS.
   • Nephritic syndrome/nephrotic syndrome.
   • Arthritis.
   • Myocarditis/pericarditis.
   • Pancreatitis/orchitis.
c. Varicella vaccine can be given for 5 years old sister within 3 to 5 days after exposure if she has not been infected or vaccinated earlier. If mother has not been infected or vaccinated earlier, VZIG can be given to the mother to prevent her from getting chicken pox but she has to be told that it may

not prevent the fetus from being infected or prevent development of total embryopathy.

A 19:

a. Congenital varicella syndrome.
b. • Shortened/malformed extremities.
   • Zigzag scarring of skin—cicatrix.
   • Neurological defects including dysfunction of anal and urethral sphincters.
   • Developmental defect of eye including Horner's syndrome and cataracts.
c. Around 25% fetus may be infected although clinically apparent disease may be seen in about 2% of fetuses whose mother had varicella in first 20 weeks of pregnancy.

A 20:

• Zidovudine.
• Lamivudine.
• Ritonavir/Nelfinavir.

For prophylaxis:
• Azithromycin—(20 mg/kg once a week or 5 mg/kg/day) for MAC prophylaxis.
• Cotrimoxazole—(150 to 750 mg/m^2/day in 2 divided doses).

A 21:

a. Class III bite.
b. i. Soap and running water for 10 minutes.
   ii. Viricidal agent (betadine).
   iii. Antimicrobial agent.
   iv. Tetanus toxoid if indicated.
   v. RIG 20 U/kg locally as much as possible (class III).
   vi. Avoid suturing.
   vii. Vaccine—0,3,7,14,30,90 (optional).

A 22:

a. Orbital cellulitis.
b. *H. influenzae, Staph. aureus*, group A beta hemolytic streptococci, *Streptococcus pneumonia* and anaerobic bacteria.
c. • Visual loss due to optic nerve involvement.
   • Cavernous sinus thrombosis.
   • Meningitis and brain abscess.

A 23:

a. Intestinal giardiasis.
b. Three stool examinations on alternate days detects around 90% of cases.
c. Metronidazole is the treatment of choice × 5 days and others are albendazole, furazolidine.

A 24:

a. Kala Azar (LD bodies-Amastigote form, nonflagellated form).
b. NNN media (Novy, MacNeil and Nicolle).
c. Amphotericin B, pentamidine, aminosidine, miltefosine, recombinant INF gamma, allopurinol and adjunct splenectomy.

A 25:

a. Such a baby has a 30% chance of getting the infection. If the mother is also HBeAg positive, the risk rises to 80–90%.
b. The baby should be given the first dose of hepatitis B vaccine within 24 hours of birth. Hepatitis B immune globulin (HBIG) preferably should also be given to the baby on the other thigh simultaneously. This is then followed by 2 more doses of the vaccine at 6 and 14 weeks or at 6 weeks and 6 months of age.
c. Yes, the baby can be found to be infected in spite of proper management if the baby has already acquired the infection in utero.
d. Once infected, 90% of the newborns become chronic carriers and 30% of them go on to develop complications like chronic hepatitis, cirrhosis and hepatocellular carcinoma.

A 26:

a. *Leishmania donovani*. Amastigote form of *Leishmania donovani* present inside macrophages in the bone marrow.
b. Sodium stibogluconate IM/IV 20 mg/kg/day for 30 days.
c. Pentamidine isethionate, amphotericin B, miltefosine.

A 27:

a. Japanese encephalitis.
b. Bites of *Culex* mosquitoes.
c.   i. JE IgM in CSF.
    ii. 4 fold or greater rise in paired sera (acute and convalescent) through IgM/IgG ELISA, HI, neutralization test.
    iii. Detection of virus antigen or genome in tissue, blood or other body fluid by immunochemistry, immunofluorescence or PCR.
    iv. Isolation- tissue culture, infant mice.
d. IgM ELISA is the method of choice.

A 28:

a. Kawasaki disease.
b. Thrombocytosis.
c. 1–3%.
d. Intravenous immunoglobulin 2 g/kg over 10–12 hours.

A 29:

a. GBS/Ac intermittent porphyria/hypokalemia.
b. Ac intermittent porphyria.

c. Urine for porphobilinogen.

d. Intravenous hemin, combined with symptomatic and supportive measures, is the treatment of choice for most acute attacks of porphyria. Mild attacks, without severe manifestations such as paresis and hyponatremia, may be treated initially with intravenous glucose.

A 30:

a. (i) HUS (ii) AGN (iii) Dyseletrcrolytemia.

b. Hyponatremia/hypernatremia/hyperkalemia.

c. IVF (ARF regime), peritoneal dialysis.

A 31:

a. HS purpura.

b. Intussusception.

c. Steroids.

A 32:

a. Pulmonary hemosiderosis.

b. Bronchoalveolar lavage showing hemosiderin laden macrophages.

c. Mitral stenosis.

A 33:

a.	Desferoxamine	—	Iron
b.	N-Acetyl cysteine	—	Acetaminophen
c.	Pyridoxine	—	Isoniazid
d.	Vitamin K	—	Coumarin
e.	BAL	—	Heavy metals (mercury, gold, arsenic)
f.	Methylene blue	—	Nitrates/methemoglobinemia
g.	Atropine	—	Organophosphate
h.	Flumazenil	—	Benzodiazepine

A 34:

a. A ring enhancing hypodense lesion seen in left frontal region with edema in bilateral frontal region.

b. Cerebral abscess.

c. When causative organism is unknown, a combination of vancomycin, 3rd generation cephalosporin and metronidazole is commonly used, usually for 4–6 weeks.

d. Surgery is indicated when:
   - Abscess > 2.5 cm in diameter.
   - Gas present in abscess.
   - Lesion is multiloculated.
   - Lesion located in posterior fossa.
   - Presence of fungus.

A 35:

a. Stevens-Johnson syndrome.
b. Antibiotics (esp. sulfonamides) and viral infection.
c. Eye—conjunctivitis, corneal ulceration, uveitis, stomatitis with ulceration, urethritis.

A 36:

a. Scabies and *Sarcoptes scabei* (Mite).
b. Application of permethrin 5% cream or 1% lindane cream or lotion to the entire body from the neck down, with particular attention to intensely involved areas, is standard therapy. The medication is left on the skin for 8–12 hour. If necessary, it may be reapplied in 1 week for another 8–12 hour period. For infants younger than 2 months, alternative therapy includes 6% sulfur in petrolatum applied for 3 consecutive 24 hour periods.

A 37:

a. Acute symptomatic giardiasis (Asymptomatic carriage form is the most common form).
b. At least 3 stool specimen collected on alternate days (Detection rate up to 90%) because there is intermittent shedding of giardial cyst.
c. Microscopy of duodenal aspirate, duodenal biopsy, fecal ELISA for antigen detection.
d. Metronidazole, albendazole, tinidazole, furazolidine and quanicrine.

A 38:

a. Epstein-Barr virus (EBV) infection (infectious mononucleosis).
b. Assay for heterophil antibodies (Monospot).
c. Symptomatic care, avoidance of contact sports while the spleen is enlarged (usually 1–3 months).
d. Acute illness lasts 2 to 4 weeks, with gradual recovery; splenic rupture is a rare but potentially fatal complication. Rarely, some patients have persistent fatigue.

Chapter
9

Neurology

Q1. Write eight distinguishing features between gray and white matter diseases of brain.

Q2. A 4-year-old boy is brought by the parents with history that the school has complained that he is aggressive, cannot sit in one place, is forgetful, restless and constantly getting into fights with his friends. At home, the parents say that he is constantly on the move and even does not watch the television continuously for more than a few minutes. The child had a normal birth and developmental milestones.

a. What is the diagnosis?
b. Give three cardinal features of this condition.
c. Name two treatment options.

Q3. A three-year-old male child is brought to you by the mother with the concern that he has been having trouble running and keeping up with his peers. She also states that he had been slow attaining other major motor milestones like walking and climbing stairs. The child is in the exam room sitting on the floor. You ask him to get up and he proceeds to arise by using his arms to climb up his legs and body.

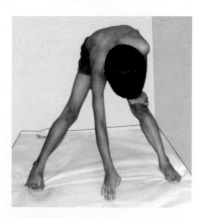

a. Name the sign.
b. Name three conditions in which this sign can be seen.
c. Name three investigations in sequence of importance.
d. What is the mode of inheritance and the locus of abnormal gene in the most common cause for this condition?

Q4. Parents bring a 1½-year-old infant for routine evaluation. He is thriving well and gross and fine motor milestones are normal for his age. The parents are concerned that the child has not started speaking as yet. A previously consulted pediatrician diagnosed the child to be autistic. On further questioning and examination, the infant is not using bisyllables like 'mama' and 'dada'. He started cooing, laughing, and babbling at the appropriate ages, but the babbling is disappearing now. He responds to a command with gestures. The child interacts with his parents and asks for objects by pointing to them. He was born at 32 weeks of gestation, and required care in the NICU, during which he received a course of antibiotics and phototherapy.

a. What is the likely diagnosis?
b. Do you agree with the diagnosis of autism? Justify your answer.
c. What is your assessment? Name two significant points in the history that could suggest an etiology for your diagnosis.
d. What investigations will you do on the child?

Q5. A 6-year-old boy and his parents come for an evaluation of a "behavioral problem". The child's teacher insists that he needs medical consultation because he is very disruptive in class. He keeps running out of class and does not concentrate on his classwork. She also states that he is careless in his work, has difficulty waiting his turn in group situations and talks excessively. The parents feel that he is just an active boy with "a lot of curiosity". They state that he can watch TV for a long period of time without problems and that other children have trouble playing with him because he "likes to be the leader". He is an only child.

a. Is the child normal? If not, what is he suffering from?
b. Name three clinical subtypes of this condition.
c. Name three drugs used in the management of this condition.

Q6. A 4-month-old baby is brought with delayed developmental milestones. Clinically, the infant is alert, interacting with the examiner and mother. Neurological examination shows the infant to be floppy with generalized hypotonia affecting the trunk and limbs. Deep tendon jerks are not elicited and there is CTEV of the left foot. Fasciculations are noted on the tongue.

a. What is the most likely diagnosis?
b. Name two definitive diagnostic tests for this condition.
c. What is the mode of inheritance in this condition?
d. Give 4 subtypes of this diagnosis.

Q7. A 4-month-old male infant, born of a consanguineous marriage to a primigravida mother, is brought to hospital with delayed milestones and feeding difficulty since birth. Antenatal period was uneventful, except that the mother did not perceive strong fetal movements. There was also history of polyhydramnios. Clinically, there is generalized hypotonia, with absent deep tendon jerks. The testes are undescended. Rest of the systemic examination is normal.

a. What would be the probable diagnosis?
b. Name 3 specific types of this disease.
c. What is the basic pathology causing this condition?
d. What would be the line of management for this child?

Q8. An 8-month-old infant is brought to hospital with complaints of excessive irritability, high-grade fever, vomiting and altered sensorium since past 18 hours. The infant had a generalized seizure 15 minutes ago. Clinical and laboratory investigations confirm meningitis. The microbiology laboratory returns the report of *H. influenza* meningitis on CSF. The child's paternal grandfather, under treatment for multiple myeloma, resides in the same house.

a. What is the prognostic significance of seizures in bacterial meningitis?
b. The commonest sequalae of bacterial meningitis is_____.
c. What would be your advice to the child's parents regarding prevention of spread of this disease to other members in the household?
d. Define household contact.

Q9. A 3-year-old female has been brought with history of low-grade fever for 2 weeks with headache, lethargy and projectile vomiting. Today she had a focal tonic-clonic seizure with loss of consciousness. She was earlier on treatment for a heart condition. Clinically, the child is comatose, febrile and her blood pressure is normal. A harsh pan systolic murmur is heard best at left sternal border. Fundus examination reveals bilateral papilledema. Reflexes are exaggerated on the left side of the body and the left plantar reflex is extensor.

a. What is the most probable diagnosis?
b. What is the etiological agent most likely responsible for the child's neurological condition? What is the likely cardiac condition?
c. What investigation would confirm the neurological diagnosis?
d. What is the first line treatment?
e. Is surgery required for the neurological disorder? List the indications for surgical intervention.

Q10. Male infant aged 7-month-old was brought with history of delayed developmental milestones and increased precordial activity, noted since 3 months of age. Clinically, the infant had tachycardia, bounding pulses, blood pressure 104/36 mm Hg, head circumference of 51 cm, with evidence of UMN involvement of the lower limbs. Cardiac examination revealed an ill sustained heaving apex in the left fifth intercostal space in the midclavicular line. Heart sounds were normal and no murmur was heard. Liver was palpable 4.5 cm below the costal margin. MR angiography is shown below.

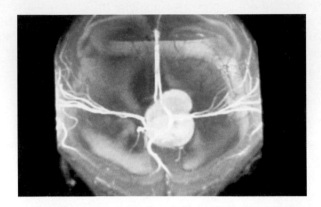

a. What is the most likely cause of the large head?
b. What clinical sign (not mentioned above) would give a clue to the diagnosis?
c. Name three signs seen on plain radiograph of the skull in hydrocephalus.
d. Name six causes of a large head.

Q11. Female neonate aged 3 days, born at home following an unbooked pregnancy to a primigravida mother was brought to the hospital with a mass on the back. Clinically, a reddish leaking lesion was seen on the lumbar region. The lower limbs were hypotonic and areflexic and the anal opening was patulous. There was a constant dribble of urine. Response to painful stimuli could not be elicited below the level of L1. Craniospinal MRI ruled out the presence of hydrocephalus.

a. What is the recurrence risk of this lesion in the next child? If a mother has had two such children in the past, what is the recurrence risk?
b. Name the drug and dosage schedule required to prevent the recurrence of this lesion in the next pregnancy.
c. The long-term neurological outlook for the neonate, in case of successful surgery is likely to be:
   i. Ambulant.
   ii. Ambulant on crutches.
   iii. Wheel chair bound.
   iv. Bedridden.
d. Name the associated central nervous system defect which may be present and name its components.

Q12. A two-year-old, previously asymptomatic child is rushed to the emergency department with history of loss of consciousness and generalized tonic, clonic seizures lasting for 2 minutes. The child had been having running nose since one day and high-grade fever since 4 hours. Clinically, the child is drowsy, with no neck stiffness, rash, or neurological deficit. Other than a congested throat, rest of the clinical examination is normal.

a. What is the indication for doing a lumbar puncture in such a case?
b. For recurrent febrile seizures, which of the following have been proved to prevent recurrence of febrile seizures: (you may select more than one answer).
   i. Antipyretics at the time of fever.
   ii. Long-term phenytoin.
   iii. Long-term carbamazepine.
   iv. Long-term phenobarbitone.
   v. Oral diazepam at the time of fever.
c. What are the diagnostic criteria for complex febrile seizures?
d. Name three factors associated with increased risk of recurrence of febrile seizures.

Q13. A 7 ½-year-old girl is brought with history that she has started having episodes of inattentiveness since 2 weeks. The episodes last 10 to 15 seconds and occur several times a day. There is no history of fall, convulsive movements, tongue bite or bladder/bowel incontinence during these periods.

a. What is your diagnosis?
b. Name one biochemical test to differentiate true seizure from a pseudoseizure.
c. Name one maneuver that is likely to precipitate the episode.
d. What is the characteristic EEG finding in this disorder?

Q14. A 6½-year-old boy is brought by his parents with the history that since the past six months, the child has undergone a marked behavioral change, with inattention, irritability, poor attention span and loss of scholastic skills. In addition, the child has stopped talking and is barely able to communicate his needs with gestures. The child was diagnosed as having autism by a doctor. Three months back, the child started having falls, which caused injuries to his face and hands, and in the past one week, has had two generalized tonic clonic seizures. Clinically, there is no nutritional or clinical abnormality noted on examination. MRI of the brain is normal.

a. What is the most likely diagnosis?
b. What is the diagnostic test for this condition?
c. What is the drug of choice for this condition?
d. What other medications can be used?

Q15. A 10-year-old girl is brought with history of gradual loss of interest in studies, psychological withdrawal, irritability, and episodes of abnormal behavior starting about 8 months back. **Treatment from various doctors and faith healers failed to provide any relief and the child started having frequent falls and involuntary, jerky movements of the limbs and trunk. These became so frequent over the past three months and now the child is completely bedridden. Clinically, the child is afebrile, normotensive, with no pallor, jaundice or cutaneous bleed. She does not respond to verbal commands. No apparent cranial nerve deficit is seen. There are involuntary movements in the form of myoclonic jerks of the trunk. Tone is increased in all four limbs (lead pipe rigidity) and deep tendon reflexs are poorly elicited.**

a. What is the likely diagnosis?
b. Name three diagnostic tests for the condition.
c. What treatment options have been studied in this condition?

Q16. A male infant aged 18-month-old is brought with history of regression of milestones and generalized seizures since the age of 1 year. The infant was well till one year of age but is now losing milestones in all sectors of development. Birth history is normal and there has been no major illness prior to one year of age. Clinically, the infant is irritable, resists handling, is pale, with few petechial spots on the abdomen and limbs. The liver is enlarged 12 cm below the costal margin and the spleen 6 cm below the costal margin. Neurologically, there is no focal deficit. Hearing, vision, fundus examination are normal. A bone marrow examination shows the presence of PAS positive staining cells.

a. What is the most probable diagnosis?
b. Other than bone marrow examination, what is the diagnostic modality?
c. What is the possible treatment and definitive cure?

Q17. A 4½-year-old girl from Gorakhpur (Eastern UP) is brought with high-grade fever with headache of 5 days duration and altered sensorium since 2 days. Several other cases have been reported from her neighborhood recently. Since this morning, the child has had three generalized tonic clonic seizures. Clinically, the child is febrile, normotensive and has mild pallor. Neurological examination reveals bilateral sixth nerve palsy, dystonia and a coarse tremor of both upper limbs.

a. What is the most likely diagnosis?
b. Name the main transmitter of this disease to man.
c. How will you reach a diagnosis of the etiology?
d. What is the preventive measure?

Q18. A 12-year-old boy is brought with history of progressive slurring of speech and frequent falls and clumsiness since the past 8 months. There is history of jaundice 2 years ago, that lasted for 2 months. Clinically, the child is pale, with hepatomegaly (5 cm below the costal margin). There is no jaundice or cutaneous bleed. Neurological examination shows presence

of dystonia, intention tremor and dysarthria. Other systems are normal. Examination of his asymptomatic younger sister who is 6 years old, reveals hepatomegaly of 4 cm, without jaundice.

a. What is the most probable diagnosis?
b. What is the pattern of inheritance?
c. What is the test to confirm the diagnosis?
d. Name two ocular findings in this disease.
e. Name the drug and dosage used in this disease.

Q19. A mother brings her 14-month-male infant with history of regression of all milestones since the past two months, following a diarrheal illness. The infant is exclusively milk fed, both from the breast and cow's milk. Clinically, the infant is conscious, pale, plump, and has sparse brownish scalp hair. Cranial nerves are normal. There is a coarse tremor of the upper and lower limbs, which disappears during sleep and a bleating cry. There is mild spasticity of all four limbs and plantars are upgoing. The MRI shows cortical atrophy.

a. What is the diagnosis?
b. What is the likely peripheral smear finding?
c. What is the treatment?

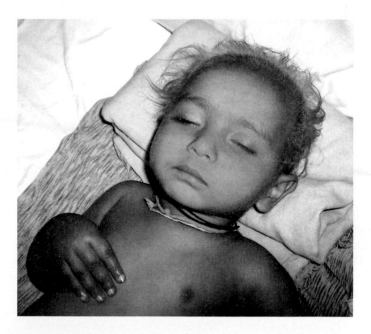

Q20. 13-year-old girl is brought with history of weakness of both the lower limbs since 3 days. Initially mild, the weakness has progressed over the past three days and the child is unable to take even a few steps and is completely bedridden. There is history of diarrhea about a month back. Clinically, the child has weakness of the lower limbs and trunk with areflexia. There is no sensory deficit but the calves and thighs are tender. Upper limbs and cranial nerves are normal.

a. What is the most probable diagnosis?
b. What is the diagnostic test for the disorder? What are the findings (give criteria).
c. What is the drug of choice and what are the indications for its use? Give the dosage schedule.

Q21. A 14-year-old boy has sustained injury to the neck due to a diving accident in the swimming pool. He is breathing on his own but cannot move or feel his arms or legs.

a. What is the recommended maneuver for opening the airway in neck injuries?
b. X-ray of the cervical spine shows no bony injury. Is it still possible for the child to have a spinal cord injury? Name the condition, its incidence and mode of diagnosis.
c. What is the emergency drug treatment that can be offered to this child?

Q22. A nine-month-old boy is taken to the Primary Health Center for a checkup and routine immunization. By mistake, the nurse gives the infant 5 mL (500,000 units) of vitamin A. One week later, the infant is brought back with features of vomiting and irritability. There is no history of fever or alteration in level of consciousness. Clinically, the physician finds a conscious infant with normal vitals, with a bulging fontanel and widening of sutures. There is no focal neurological deficit and rest of the examination is essentially normal.

a. What is the most probable diagnosis?
b. What findings do you expect the CSF to show?
c. Name three drugs that can lead to a similar clinical situation.
d. Name one complication of this disease.

Q23. A previously well, 3½-year-old girl comes with history of sudden onset of unsteadiness while walking since 4 days. Initially, the complaint was mild but now the child is unable to walk and is reluctant to sit up in bed. There is history of fever with a rash about 2 weeks back. Clinically, the child is afebrile, normotensive, and has no neck stiffness or features of raised intracranial pressure. The cranial nerves are normal. The child has truncal ataxia. Tone is diminished in all the four limbs and there is nystagmus with fast component to the right, with past pointing, and dysarthria.

a. What is the most probable diagnosis?
b. Is there a role of CSF examination in this child? What findings do you expect?
c. What is the likely organism responsible?

Q24. This 7½-year-old girl was brought with history of delayed developmental milestones and generalized seizures. As an infant she had had myoclonic seizures.

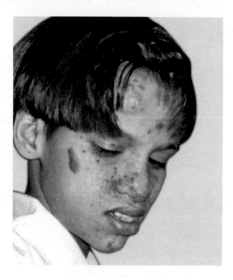

a. What is the diagnosis? What are the lesions on the face?
b. Name three other types of skin lesions seen in this condition.
c. What is the inheritance?
d. Name three organ systems other than skin and brain that may be affected.

Q25. Study the image of the 10-year-old child and answer the questions.

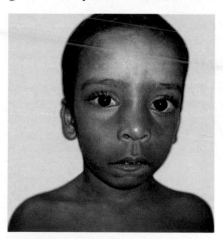

a. Name the lesion and the syndrome that it forms a part of.
b. What are the neurological morbidities of this syndrome (Name three).
c. What is the ocular complication that can accompany?
d. Name the radiological sign associated with cranial involvement.

Q26. A 2½-year-old child is brought by the mother with history of poor development of speech. The child plays with his toys but not with other children. He also does not respond to her calls. On examination, the motor system, sensory system, hearing and vision are normal. The child is able to say a few words. He does not interact with the examiner.

a. What is the most probable diagnosis?
b. What are the three characteristic features of this condition?
c. Which part of the brain is affected in this condition?
d. What is the scale used to assess this condition?

Q27. Match the following.

1. Chorea   A. Rhythmic, oscillatory movement caused by simultaneous contractions of antagonistic muscles
2. Athetosis   B. Brief flexion contraction of a muscle group, resulting in a sudden jerk
3. Dystonia   C. Rapid, unsustained, irregular, purposeless, nonpatterned movement
4. Tremor   D. Slow, coarse, writhing movement that is more pronounced in the distal muscles
5. Myoclonus   E. Sustained, slow, twisting motion that may progress to a fixed posture and can be activated by repetitive movement

Q 28.   Study the plain CT scan film of a breastfed 3-month-old infant who was brought to the hospital with history of left-sided focal seizures.

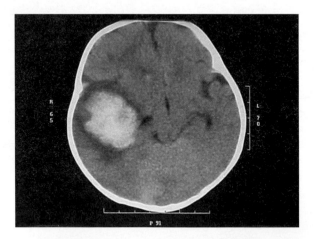

a. What is the CT scan finding suggestive of and what is the most probable diagnosis?
b. How would you confirm the etiological diagnosis? Name three tests.
c. What is the preventive measure for this condition?

ANSWERS

A 1:

Gray matter disease	White matter disease
Dementia: Early	Late
Seizures: Early prominent	Late
Disturbed tone, gait, reflexes : Uncommon late	Most prominent feature
Basal ganglia signs symptoms: Present	Absent
Retinitis pigmentosa: May be present	Absent
MRI: Cortical atrophy, basal ganglia disease	Good yield for white matter disease
ERG: May be abnormal	Normal
VER/BERA: Normal	Abnormal

A 2:

a. Attention deficit hyperactivity disorder.
b. Inattention, hyperactivity and impulsivity.
c. • Medications (methyl phenidate, amphetamines, fluoxitine, atomoxi-tine)
   • Behavior therapy.

A 3:

a. Gower's sign.
b. Duchenne muscular dystrophy, spinal muscular atrophy type III, limb girdle dystrophy, Becker muscular dystrophy, myopathy.
c. Dystrophin gene study, electromyograph/nerve conduction velocity, Creatinine phosphokinase levels.
d. X-linked recessive/Xp 21 (for DMD).

A 4:

a. Hearing loss.
b. No. The child is interacting with parents, pointing at objects.
c. The infant has hearing loss. The significant points in the history include the antibiotics received (aminoglycosides), and bilirubin-induced brain injury. Other factors could be meningitis, prematurity, excessive noise in NICU (not mentioned in question).
d. Play audiometry, BERA, impedence audiometry.

A 5:

a. Attention deficit hyperactivity disorder.
b.   i. Attention—deficit/hyperactivity disorder, predominantly inattentive type.
    ii. Attention—deficit/hyperactivity disorder, predominantly hyperactive-impulsive type.
    ii. Attention—deficit/hyperactivity disorder, combined type.
c. Methyl phenidate, amphetamines, fluoxitine, atomoxitine.

A 6:

a. Spinal muscular atrophy type I (Werdnig Hoffman disease).
b. Electromyography, muscle biopsy, genetic analysis for SMN gene.
c. Autosomal recessive.
d. Type I—severe infantile form (Werdnig Hoffman disease).
   Type II—late infantile and more slowly progressive.
   Type III—chronic or juvenile form (Kugelberg Welander disease).
   Type 0—severe fetal form; usually lethal in utero.

A 7:

a. Congenital myopathy.
b. Myotubular myopathy.
   Nemaline rod myopathy.
   Central core disease.
c. Maturational arrest of fetal muscle during myotubular stage of development.
d. (i) Confirm the disease, (ii) Physiotherapy, (iii) NG feeds, (iv) Genetic counseling.

A 8:

a. Prognosis related to generalized seizure depends upon time of onset and duration. Seizures persisting after 4 days into the course of meningitis and which are difficult to treat have poor neurological prognosis.
b. Sensorineural hearing loss.
c. Rifampicin prophylaxis for family members @ 20 mg/kg (max 600 mg) once daily for 4 days for all household members.
d. Household contact: A household contact is one who lives in the residence of the index case or who has spent a minimum of 4 hours with the index case for at least 5 of the 7 days preceding the patient's hospitalization.

A 9:

a. Cerebral abscess (right sided).
b. *Streptococcus pyogenes* (Group A, B) *S. milleri, S. pneumonia, S. fecalis.* Cyanotic heart disease with right to left shunt.
c. Contrast CT scan or MRI head.
d. In the presence of cyanotic congenital heart disease: ampicillin + sulbactam with or without metronidazole + 3rd generation cephalosporin.
e. CT guided aspiration if: encapsulated abscess, raised intracranial pressure, mass effect. Surgical excision if: Abscess > 2.5 cm in diameter, gas in abscess, multiloculated lesion, lesion in posterior fossa, fungus isolated from abscess.

A 10:

a. Vein of Galen malformation.
b. Cranial bruit on auscultation.
c. (i) Sutural separation (ii) Erosion of the posterior clinoid process (iii) Beaten silver appearance (increase in convolutional markings).
d. (i) Rickets (ii) Osteogenesis imperfect (iii) Epiphyseal dysplasia (iv) Chronic subdural hematoma/effusion (v) Megalencephaly due to Tay-Sachs disease,

gangliosidosis, mucopolysaccharidosis (vi) Aminoacidurias (maple syrup urine disease) (vii) Leucodystrophies (metachromatic leucodystrophy, Alexander disease, Canavan disease) (viii) Cerebral gigantism (ix) Familial megalencephaly (x) Chronic anemia.

A 11:

a. 3–4%, 10%.
b. Folic acid, 4 mg daily beginning one month prior to planned conception.
c. Wheelchair bound.
d. Chiari defect type II—Herniation of cerebellar inferior vermis, pons and medulla through foramen magnum, hydrocephalus, elongation of 4th ventricle, kinking of brainstem.

A 12:

a. Lumbar puncture should be performed if:
   i. The infant is less than 12 months of age.
   ii. Consider LP if the infant is between 12 and 18 months of age and seizures are complex or sensorium remains clouded.
   iii. Meningitis cannot be excluded on clinical grounds.
b. (iv,v) Long-term phenobarbitone and oral diazepam at the time of fever.
c. Complex partial seizures:
   i. Duration > 15 minutes.
   ii. Repeated convulsions in 24 hours.
   iii. Focal seizure activity or focal findings during the postictal stage.
d. Factors associated with increased risk of recurrence.
   i. Age < 12 months.
   ii. Lower temperature at onset of seizures.
   iii. Positive family history of febrile seizures.
   iv. Complex febrile seizures.

A 13:

a. Simple absence seizure.
b. Serum prolactin level will be increased in a true seizure but not in a pseudoseizure.
c. Hyperventilation for 3–4 minutes.
d. 3 per second spike and wave pattern.

A 14:

a. Landau Kleffner syndrome.
b. EEG: shows high amplitude spike and wave discharges, more apparent during non-REM sleep.
c. Valproate is the drug of choice.
d. Clobazam, steroids.

A 15:

a. Subcaute scleorsing panencephalitis.
b. i. CSF measles antibody titer > 1: 8, ii. EEG: Burst suppression pattern, iii. Isolation of virus or viral antigen on brain biopsy.
c. Isoprinosine, interferon $\alpha_2\beta$.

A 16:

a. Gaucher disease.
b. β-glucosidase enzyme levels in leucocytes, cultured fibroblasts.
c. Enzyme replacement therapy (60U/alternate week) with recombinant acid β-glucosidase (imiglucerase). Bone marrow transplantation is the definitive cure.

A 17:

a. Japanese encephalitis.
b. Female culex mosquito *(Culex tritaeniorhynchus* and *C.vishnui).*
c. i. JE IgM in CSF, ii. 4 fold or greater rise in IgM/IgG, HI or neutralization tests in paired sera (acute and convalescent), iii. Detection of virus antigen or genome in tissue, blood or other body fluid by immunochemistry, immunofluorescence or PCR, iv. Isolation-tissue culture, infant mice.
d. Vaccine in the interepidemic stage and fogging with malathion in 3 km range from the infected case.

A 18:

a. Wislon disease.
b. Autosomal recessive.
c. Hepatic copper content (>250 µg/g dry weight of liver).
d. Kayser-Fleischer ring, sunflower cataract.
e. D penicillamine 20 mg/kg/day in two divided doses.

A 19:

a. Infantile tremor syndrome.
b. Macrocytic anemia.
c. Vitamin $B_{12.}$

A 20:

a. Guillain Barre syndrome, postinfectious polyneuropathy.
b. CSF: Albuminocytological dissociation. CSF protein more than twice the normal level and cells < 10/cumm.
c. Intravenous immunoglobulin, rapidly progressive paralysis, 400 mg/kg/day × 5 days.

A 21:

a. Jaw thrust without head tilt.
b. Yes, SCIWORA (spinal cord injury without radiographic (bone) abnormalities), lucidence (20%), MRI of the spine.
c. High dose methyl prednisolone within 8 hours of injury.

A 22:

a. Pseudotumor cerebri.
b. Normal.
c. Nalidixic acid, doxycycline, minocycline, tetracycline, nitrofurantoin, isotretinoin.
d. Optic atrophy, blindness.

A 23:

a. Acute cerebellar ataxia.
b. CSF would show mild increase in protein, and pleocytosis, without abnormalities of sugar or culture.
c. Varicella.

A 24:

a. Tuberous sclerosis, adenoma sebaceum.
b. Hypopigmented macules, shagreen patch, periungual fibromas, subungual fibromas.
c. Autosomal dominant with variable penetrance.
d. Retinal phakomas, renal cysts, cardiac rhabdomyoma, bone cysts, rectal polyps, dental enamel pits, gingival fibromas, nonrenal hamartomas, retinal achromic patches.

A 25:

a. Prot wine stain, Sturge-Weber syndrome.
b. Seizures, hemiparesis, stroke-like episodes, mental retardation.
c. Glaucoma, buphthalmos.
d. Intracranial calcification ("Railroad track" appearance).

A 26:

a. Autistic disorder.
b. (i) Impairment in verbal and nonverbal communication, (ii) Impairment in reciprocal and social interaction, (iii) Imaginative repetitive activity.
c. Cerebellum, reticular activating system, hippocampus.
d. CARS (Childhood autism rating scale).

A 27:

Chorea	Rapid, unsustained, irregular, purposeless, nonpatterned movement
Athetosis	Slow, coarse, writhing movement that is more pronounced in the distal muscles
Dystonia	Sustained, slow, twisting motion that may progress to a fixed posture and can be activated by repetitive movement
Tremor	Rhythmic, oscillatory movement caused by simultaneous contractions of antagonistic muscles
Myoclonus	Brief flexion contraction of a muscle group, resulting in a sudden jerk

A 28:

a. Intracranial hemorrhage right temporoparietal region with midline shift. Late onset vitamin K dependant bleeding (late onset hemorrhagic disease of the newborn).
b. Abnormal PT, abnormal APTT, raised PIVKA.
c. Injection vitamin K 1 mg intramuscular at birth to every baby.

Neonatal Advanced Life Support and Pediatric Advanced Life Support

QUESTIONS

Q1. NRP Chart

- Enlists 5 points in routine care of newborn.

Q2. Positive pressure ventilation

a. Enlist 3 common problems encountered in PPV
b. Mention or demonstrate the techniques to improve PPV using bag and mask if above problems are encountered.

Q3. Fill in the blanks

Weight (g)	Gestational age (wks)	ET Tube size (mm) (inside diameter)	Suction Catheter Size(F)
Below 1000	Below 28	?	?
1000–2000	28–34	?	?
2000–3000	34–38	?	?
Above 3000	Above 38	?	?

Q4.

a. What is the recommended dose of biphasic energy to be delivered by AED?
b. True false
   As per recent ILCOR 2010
   i. Cuffed tracheal tube are unsafe and ineffective in pediatric population
   ii. Pulse check is de-emphasized
   iii. Look listen and feel step is removed
c. Fill in the blanks
   i. VF and VT contribute to_____% pediatric cardiac arrest
   ii. Major cause of pediatric cardiac arrest is_____.
   iii. ILCOR stands for_____.
   iv. ABC is changed to_____.
d. What is the ideal depth and rate of pediatric CPR?

Q5. A term baby is born by normal vaginal delivery. Amniotic fluid was not stained with meconium. The baby is born limp and is not crying. Resuscitate with the provided dummy and equipment. You are free to ask vital signs of the baby whenever appropriate.

Q6. You are resuscitating a newborn at birth. The baby has gasping respiration at 30 seconds after birth. Demonstrate what steps you would take for the next 30 seconds.

Q7. You are resuscitating a newborn at birth. The baby is limp and blue, heart rate <100. You have done following steps: Warmed and positioned, suctioned, dried, stimulated, given bag and mask ventilation (40–60/min). Heart rate was <60/min and cardiac massage was given (120/min) along with bag and tube ventilation (due to inadequate bag and mask ventilation). There was no improvement. Demonstrate what steps you would take for the resuscitation of this newborn.

Q8. You have been called to attend a call from the operation theatre of a primi mother with a 35 weeks IUGR baby. Mother has PIH and now the fetus has developed fetal bradycardia and Doppler studies show absent flows in MCA. Half an hour ago there was meconium staining of the amniotic fluid. How will you proceed on reaching the operation theatre? What are the actions you will take in the first 60 seconds?

Q9. Calculate the size of cuffed and uncuffed tube required for a 4-years-old child who requires intubation. Also calculate the depth of insertion of the tube. Give the formulae used.

Q10. Write the possible routes of administration of the following drugs (write "yes" or "no" in the appropriate box to signify that the drug can be given by that route).

Sl. No.	Drugs	Intravenous	Intraosseous	Intratracheal
a.	Lignocaine			
b.	Epinephrine			
c.	Atropine			
d.	Naloxone			
e.	Sodium bicarbonate			
f.	Adenosine			
g.	Dopamine			
h.	Calcium gluconate			

Q11. A 9-year-old boy is brought to the emergency in a pulseless state. ECG shows electrical activity suggestive of ventricular tachycardia.
a. Name 8 etiologies that can precipitate pulseless electrical activity.
b. What is the dose at which defibrillation is initiated?
c. Name three drugs that can be used if defibrillation and adrenaline fail.
d. What is the ratio of cardiac compression to breathing prior to and after intubation and initiation of IPPR?

Q12. The following are complications related to hypothermia except:

a. Ventricular fibrillation.

b. ARDS.

c. Hyperglycemia.

d. Thrombocytosis.

Q13. A 14-month-old baby is brought with history of choking while playing with some beads. On arrival he has an inspiratory stridor, and suprasternal retractions. Chest rise and air entry are poor. Demonstrate five initial actions that you will perform.

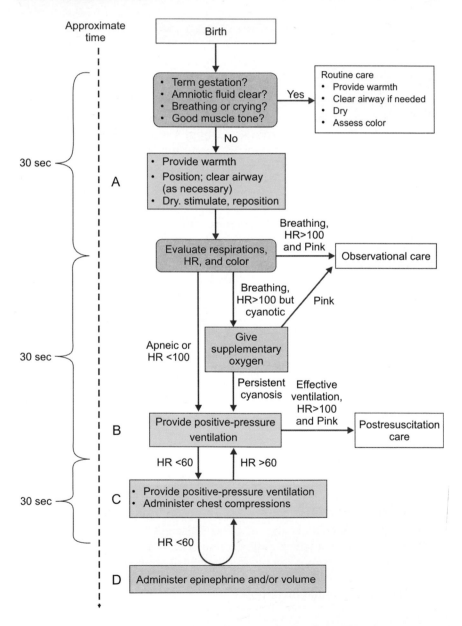

ANSWERS

A 1:

- Dry baby on mother's abdomen
- Provide warmth (skin to skin care)
- Assure open airway if needed
- Cut cord in 1–2 minutes
- Ongoing evaluation of neonate.

A 2:

a. Inadequate seal
   Inappropriate position
   Blocked airway
   Inadequate pressure
b. Techniques to improve PPV using bag and mask.

Inadequate seal	**M**ask adjusted to ensure airtight seal
Inappropriate position	**R**eposition the head in sniffing position
Blocked airway	**S**uction the airway **O**pen baby's mouth and ventilate
Inadequate pressure	Increase **P**ressure by squeezing the bag with more pressure till a chest rise is visible
No improvement with above steps	**A**lternate airway-Consider endotracheal intubation

A 3:

Weight (g)	Gestational age (wks)	ET Tube size (mm) (inside diameter)	Suction Catheter Size(F)
Below 1000	Below 28	2.5	5F or 6F
1000–2000	28–34	3.0	6F or 8F
2000–3000	34–38	3.5	8F
Above 3000	Above 38	3.5–4.0	8F or 10F

A 4:

a. First dose-2J/kg
   Subsequent dose-4J/kg
b.
   i. False
   ii. True
   iii. True

c.
    i. 5–15%
    ii. Asphyxia
    iii. International Liaison committee on resuscitation
    iv. CAB.
d. 100/min
   5 cm or 2 inches in child
   4 cm or 1.5 inch in infants.

A 5:

a. Mention your intention to handwash.
b. Check the equipment: Radiant warmer, oxygen source, suction, ambu bag—if time is available. If not, mention your intention to have done so prior to baby's birth.
c. Perform all basic steps within 30 seconds in correct order—Provide warmth, suction-clear airway, dry and stimulate, give O_2 if required.
d. Evaluate and ask for vitals—Examiner says HR <100/min.
e. Bag and mask ventilation—Self-inflating resuscitation bag, look for correct assembling of parts, position the baby correctly, select proper size mask. Position mask and provide appropriate ventilation (rate and rise–40-60/min). Say out loud: *squeeze-two-three-squeeze-*
f. Evaluate vitals—Examiner says HR < 60/min.
g. Mention your intention to have an assistant to provide bag and mask ventilation during chest compressions.
h. Chest compression—two finger technique, depth 1/3 of AP diameter of the chest ratio 1:3, check pulses. Say out loud: *One-and two-and three-and squeeze-and*
i. Evaluate HR decide about medication.
j. Epinephrine is indicated if HR <60 after 30 secconds of assisted ventilation and 30 seconds of coordinated chest compression and ventilations.

A 6:

a. Check Ambu bag, mask, reservoir and oxygen source.
b. Attach reservoir, and oxygen source.
c. Correct technique of ambu bagging—good seal, look for chest rise.
d. Correct frequency of ambu bagging—40–60 breaths per minute. Say out loud: *squeeze-two-three-squeeze-two-three.*
e. Count heart rate at end of 30 seconds—by applying stethoscope or palpating base of umbilical cord for 6 seconds.

A 7:

a. Place IV or umbilical line.
b. Asks if mother has received narcotics.
c. If no, then give epinephrine—0.1–0.3 mL/kg 1:10,000 IV or IT.
d. If no improvement soda bicarb 2 mEq/kg IV slowly.

e. If no improvement check that bag delivers 100% O_2.
f. Check that head is not overflexed.
g. Check that ET tube is in trachea.
h. Adequate ventilation pressure is being provided.
i. Adequate cardiac massage is being given.

A 8:

a. Check the equipment.
b. Perform all basic steps within 30 seconds in correct order—Provide warmth, suction-clear airway, dry and stimulate, give O_2 if required.
c. Evaluates and ask for vitals: Examiner says HR <100.
d. • Bag and mask ventilation self-inflating resuscitation bag.
   • Correct assembling of parts.
   • Position baby correctly.
   • Select proper sized mask.
   • Provide ventilation.
   • Check chest rise.
   • Rate of ventilation 40–60/min.
   • Evaluate vitals (HR < 60, HR > 60/min).

A 9:

a. Uncuffed: $\dfrac{\text{age in years}}{4} + 4 = \dfrac{4+4}{4} = 5.0$

b. Uncuffed: $\dfrac{\text{age in years}}{4} + 3 = \dfrac{4+3}{4} = 4.0$

c. Depth of insertion: $\dfrac{\text{age in years}}{2} + 12 = 14$ cm

A 10:

Sl. No.	Drug	Intravenous	Intraosseous	Intratracheal
a.	Lignocaine	Yes	Yes	Yes
b.	Epinephrine	Yes	Yes	Yes
c.	Atropine	Yes	Yes	Yes
d.	Naloxone	Yes	Yes	Yes
e.	Sodium bicarbonate	Yes	Yes	No
f.	Adenosine	Yes	Yes	No
g.	Dopamine	Yes	Yes	No
h.	Calcium gluconate	Yes	Yes	No

A 11:

a. Hypothermia, hypoxemia, hypovolemia, hypokalemia, hyperkalemia, metabolic disorders, cardiac tamponade, tension pneumothorax, toxins, thromboembolism.
b. 2 J/kg.
c. Amiodarone 5 mg/kg, lignocaine 1 mg/kg, magnesium sulfate 25–50 mg/kg.
d. Before intubation and initiation of IPPR: 15:2, after intubation and initiation of IPPR: 5:1.

A 12: d. Thrombocytosis.

A 13:

a. Lie the infant flat on his back.
b. Open the airway by head-tilt, chin lift maneuver.
c. Give five chest thrusts.
d. Turn the baby over on your hand and give five back blows.
e. Open the mouth and try to visualize the foreign body.

Community Medicine

QUESTIONS

Q1. What is the full form of following abbreviations of national programs?

a. IMNCI

b. NSSK

c. VHNDs

d. HBNC

e. JSY

d. JSSK

g. RBSK

Q2. National institute of nutrition.

a. Where is it located

b. Mention 2 centers working under NIN

c. State TRUE or FALSE

    i. Gives special reference to protein energy malnutrition

    ii. Was established in 1918

    iii. Had previous names as Beri-Beri' enquiry unit, deficiency disease enquiry, nutrition research laboratories.

Q3. NACO

a. Was launched in _____.

b. Provide leadership through_____HIV/AIDS prevention and control Societies

c. Year of NACP-I (_____)

d. Year of NACP-II (_____)

e. Is a division of_____.

f. What are goals and objectives of NACO-4.

Q4. UIP Significant milestones- Mention the year

a. Expanded program of immunization

b. UIP Was launched

c. Measles was launched
d. Vitamin A was launched
e. Hepatitis B was added.

Q5. Japanese Encephalitis (JE vaccine) vaccine

a. True false
    i.   Is a part of UIP
    ii. Was introduced in 112 endemic districts in campaign mode in phased manner
b. What is the most vulnerable age group ?
    i.   0–1 Year
    ii. 1–5 Year
    iii. 5–10 Year
    iv. 10–15 Years
c. Enlist 5 focus states
d. Enlist 4 states where JE Vaccination was provided in 2013–14.

Q6. Answer the following questions.

a. National Malaria Control Program (NMCP) was launched in India in_____ year.
b. National Malaria Eradication Program (NMEP) was launched in_____ year.
c. Name the four phases of NMEP.
d. Modified plan of operation under NMEP came into force from_____ year.
e. Endemic areas under modified plan of operation under NMEP is defined as annual parasite index (API) > _____.
f. Within the modified plan of operation an additional component known as "*P. falciparum* containment program" has been introduced from October 1977, through the assistance of_____ agency.

Q7. Answer the following questions.

a. When was National Tuberculosis Control Program started?
b. When was Revised National Tuberculosis Control Program started?
c. Under RNTCP treatment services will be made most assessable to the patients with a view to achieve a cure rate of at least _____% amongst all newly detected sputum positive cases.
d. In tuberculosis control program DTC stands for _____.
e. One tuberculosis unit will function as managerial unit for_____ lakh population. In tribal area, the population it caters to, is _____ lakhs.

Q8. National programs.

a. Define 'Problem Village' as described under National Water Supply and Sanitation Program.
b. Name four components of Minimum Needs Program (8 components).
c. Name the technique invented by Environmental Engineering Research Institute Nagpur for defluoridation of water.

Q9. Answer the following regarding child survival and safe motherhood program.

a. When was it initiated?
b. Name five child survival components of CSSM program.
c. Which drug does CSSM drug kit supply and for what purpose?

Q10. Yearly data (for year 2000) pertaining to deliveries and their outcome in a community is as follows.

No. of total births	:	10,000
No. of still births	:	80
No. of preterm deliveries	:	1500
No. of newborn deaths		
In first week of life	:	320
During 2 to 4 weeks of life	:	180
No. of deaths during first year of life	:	500

Calculate perinatal and neonatal mortality rates for this community, demonstrating the steps taken to arrive at the results.

Q11. Answer the following questions.

a. Name different measures practiced for ensuring enhanced child survival under the CSSM program.
b. Name prophylactic measures advocated under the National Nutritional Anemia Control Program to reduce prevalence of anemia in children.
c. What measures are practiced by health care workers to improve nutrition of children under the ICDS?

Q12. Answer the following questions regarding RNTPC.

a. What constitutes a case of relapse of tuberculosis as defined by the RNTCP?
b. Define a defaulter of treatment and a failure.
c. What is recommended management for each of these cases?

Q13. What are the goals of the National Health Policy (MCH) 2010 in terms of:

a. Infant mortality rate.
b. Under 5 mortality rate.
c. Immunization of infants.
d. Immunization of pregnant women.
e. Maternal mortality rate.

Q14.

a. Write down the composition of the meal in Mid Day Meal Program in terms of quantity of grain, calories and protein provided.
b. Give two examples of premixed foods used in this program.
c. According to National Institute of Nutrition minimum number of feeding days in a year should be _____ (mention days) to have desired impact on the children.

Q15.

a. Match new units for the older units of radiation measurement:

Old units	New units
1. Curie (C)	a. Coulombs/kg
2. Rad	b. Becquerel (Bq)
3. Rem	c. Sievert (Sv)
4. Roentgen (R)	d. Gray (Gy)

b. Black bags/bins are meant for what type of waste?
    i. Infectious waste.
    ii. Noninfectious waste like paper/glass.
    iii. Organic waste like discarded food/vegetables, etc.
    iv. Both ii and iii.
c. Name 4 syndromes with increased sensitivity to X-rays.

Q16. You are provided with.
- Bin lined with black plastic bag.
- Blue puncture proof container.
- Bin lined with yellow plastic bag.
- Bin lined with red plastic bag.

a. List which bag will you segregate for the following items:
    i. Used wound dressing material.
    ii. Syringe wrappers.
    iii. Needles.
    iv. Used indwelling umbilical catheters.
b. How will you dispose the following hospital waste?
    i. Non-infectious waste.
    ii. Infected solid waste.
    iii. Infected plastics.
    iv. Sharps.
c. What do these two symbols stand for?

Q17. Give the nutritional value (calories and protein) of following cooked items.

Sl. No.	Item (quantity)	Calories	Proteins
a.	One chapatti or one bread		
b.	One biscuit		
c.	One egg		
d.	One tsf meshed potato		
e.	One tsf cooked dal.		

Q18. Answer the following questions.

a. Dextrose content of 1 liter Ringer lactate.
b. Na^+ content of one mL of 3% NaCl.
c. Na^+ content of 100 mL of 0.9% of NaCl.
d. Elemental Ca in 1 mL of 10% calcium gluconate.
e. K^+ content of 1 liter of Isolyte-P.

Q 19. Answer the following questions.

a. Give 4 parameters for malaria surveillance under NMEP.
b. As per National Leprosy Eradication Program (NLEP), the aim is to reduce case load to less than _____ per 10,000.
c. As per RNTCP, augmentation of case finding activities through quality sputum microscopy is to detect at least ____ % of estimated cases.
d. As per RNTCP, achievement of least _____% cure rate through supervised short course chemotherapy is aimed.

Q 20. Answer the following questions.

a. When was ICDS program started?
b. Mention nutritional components of ICDS.
c. Who supervises the work of anganwadi in ICDS?
d. As per vitamin A prophylaxis schedule, what is the dose of vitamin A given to children <12 months of age and how often?

Q 21. State true/false.

a. The National School Health Program undertakes examination of school children by camp approach during 2 days on 3 consecutive months of a year.
b. National Blindness Control Program is a sponsored program.
c. All children in the age group 9 months to 3 years are administered 2 lac units of vitamin A at 6 monthly intervals as per vitamin A deficiency control program.
d. The Mid Day Meal Program is a Central Government Sponsored Program.

ANSWERS

A 1:

a. IMNCI- Integrated Management of Neo-natal and Childhood Illness
b. NSSK -Navjaat Shishu Suraksha Karyakram
c. VHNDs -Village Health and Nutrition Days
d. HBNC- Home Based Newborn Care
e. JSY-Janani Suraksha Yojana
f. JSSK-Janani Shishu Suraksha Karyakram
g. RBSK-Rashtriya Bal Swasthya Karyakram.

A 2:

a. Hyderabad
b. Food And Drug Toxicology Research Centre (FDTRC) in 1971
   National Nutrition Monitoring Bureau (NNMB) in 1972 and
   National Centre for Laboratory Animal Sciences (NCLAS) in 1976
c. True, True, True

A 3:

a. Was launched in–1992
b. Provide leadership through 35 HIV/AIDS Prevention and Control Societies
c. Year of NACP-I (1992-1999)
d. Year of NACP-II (1999-2006)
e. Is a division of the ministry of Health and Family Welfare
f. Goals and Objectives
Objective 1: Reduce new infections by 50% (2007 Baseline of NACP III)
Objective 2: Comprehensive care, support and treatment to all persons living with HIV/AIDS

A 4:

a. Expanded program of immunisation—1978
b. UIP was launched in—1985
c. Measles was launched in 1985
d. Vit A was launched in 1990
e. Hep B was added in 2007

A 5:

a. i. True
    ii. True
b. Answer b-1–5 years
c. Assam, Bihar, Tamil Nadu, Uttar Pradesh and West Bengal
d. Bihar
   Tamil Nadu
   Karnataka
   West Bengal

A 6:

a.   1953
b.   1958
c.   (i) Preparatory (ii) Attack (iii) Consolidation (iv) Maintenance.
d.   1977
e.   2
f.   Swedish International Development Agency.

A 7:

a.   1962
b.   1992
c.   85%
d.   District Tuberculosis Center.
e.   5 lakhs; 2.5 lakhs.

A 8:

a.   Problem village is one where:
    i.   No source of safe water is available within distance of 1.6 km.
    ii.   Where water is available at depth more than 15 meter.
    iii.   Water source has excess of salinity, iron, fluorides and other toxic elements.
    iv.   Water is exposed to risk of cholera.
b.   i.   Rural health.
    ii.   Rural water supply.
    iii.   Rural electrification.
    iv.   Elementary education.
    v.   Adult education.
    vi.   Nutrition.
    vii.   Environmental improvement of urban slums.
    viii.   Houses of landless laborers.
c.   Nalgonda technique.

A 9:

a.   Initiated in 1992.
b.   i.   Neonatal care.
    ii.   Immunization.
    iii.   Vitamin A deficiency control and prophylaxis.
    iv.   Diarrhea control and ORT.
    v.   ARI control and therapy.
c.   The program includes training of peripheral level health worker on recognition of pneumonia and treatment with cotrimoxazole.

A 10:

Perinatal mortality rate: $= 80 + 320/10,000 \times 1000$
$= 40$ per 1000 live births
Neonatal mortality rate: $= 320 + 180/10,000 \times 1000$
$= 50$ per 1000 live births

A 11:

a. Immunization, management of diarrhea with ORS, treatment of acute respiratory infections, vitamin A supplementation, essential newborn care.
b. Iron Folic Acid supplements for at least 100 days of the year.
   Iron—20 mg and folic acid 100 micro gram with use of iron rich foods.
c. Supplementary nutrition to provide extra calories and proteins, vitamin A supplementation and use of iodized salt in the food prepared.

A 12:

a. *Relapse:* Patient, who returns smear positive, having previously been treated for tuberculosis and declared cured after completion of his treatment.
b. *Defaulter:* Patient, who returns sputum smear positive after having left treatment for least 2 months.
   Failure: Patient, who was initially smear positive, who began treatment and who remained or became smear positive again at 5 months or later during the course of treatment.
c. Category II of RNTCP with 2 SHRZE, 1 HRZE, 5 HRE.

A 13:

a. Reduce to < 30/1000 live birth.
b. < 10/1000 live birth.
c. 100%.
d. 100%.
e. < 1/lakh.

A 14:

a. Cereals and millets   -   75 g/day/child
   Pulses   -   30 g/day/child
   Oils and fats   -   8 g/day/child
   Leafy vegetables   -   30 g/day/child
   Non leafy vegetables   -   30 g/day/child
   Food grain component 100 g per child per day or equivalent precooked food or through the supply of 5 kg wheat/rice per month per child in a family for 10 months. Provides 300 calories and 8–12 g protein per day.
b. *Shakti ahar:* Roasted wheat 40 g/roasted gram 20 g/roasted peanut 10 gm/ jaggery 30 g.
   Hyderabad mix: Whole wheat 40 g/bengal gram 16 g/groundnut 10 g/ jaggery 20 g.
c. 250 days/year. Beneficiary should attend school for 20 days/month.

A 15:

a.

Old units	New units
1. Curie (C)	Becquerel (Bq)
2. Rad	Gray (Gy)
3. Rem	Sievert (Sv)
4. Roentgen (R)	Coulombs/kg

b. (iv); Noninfectious waste like paper/glass and organic waste like discarded food/vegetables, etc.
c. Ataxia telangiectasia, Basal cell nevoid syndrome, Cockayne syndrome, Down syndrome, Fanconi anemia, Gardner syndrome, Nijmegan breakage syndrome, Usher syndrome, Bloom syndrome.

A 16:

a. i. Bin lined with yellow plastic bag.
   ii. Bin lined with black plastic bag.
   iii. Blue puncture proof container.
   iv. Bin lined with red plastic bag.
b. i. Landfill.
   ii. Incineration.
   iii. Disinfected and shred.
   iv. Mutilate with heat.
c. i. Biohazard.
   ii. Cytotoxic.

A 17:

Sl. No.	Item (quantity)	Calories	Proteins (g)
a.	One chapatti or one bread	70	2
b.	One biscuit	20	0.5
c.	One egg	80	6
d.	One tsf meshed potato	40	nil
e.	One tsf cooked dal	10	0.5

A 18:

a. Dextrose content of 1 liter Ringer lactate is zero.
b. Na^+ content of one ml of 3% NaCl is 0.5 mEq.
c. Na^+ content of 100 ml of 0.9% of NaCl is 15.4 mEq.
d. Elemental Ca in 1 ml of 10% calcium gluconate is 9 mg.
e. K^+ content of 1 liter of Isolyte-P is 20 mEq/L.

A 19:

a. i. Annual parasite index.
   ii. Annual blood examination rate.
   iii. Annual falciparum incidence.
   iv. Slide falciparum rate.
b. 1 per 10,000.
c. 70%.
d. 85%.

A 20:

a. 1961.
b. Supplementary nutrition, vitamin A prophylaxis, iron and folic acid distribution.
c. Mukhyasevikas.

d. <12 months—55 mg (1 lac IU) once every 4 to 6 months.
    >12 months—110 mg (2 lac IU) once every 4 to 6 months.

A 21:

a. False (3 days, 2 consecutive months).
b. True.
c. True.
d. False.

Respiratory System

Q1. Give position for postural drainage of both right middle lobe and lingula (left) (physiotherapy demonstration not required).

Q2. Respiratory compensation of metabolic disorders. What is the conversion factor (PCO$_2$) with each change of (HCO$_3^-$)?

Disorder

a. Metabolic acidosis
b. Metabolic alkalosis

Q3.

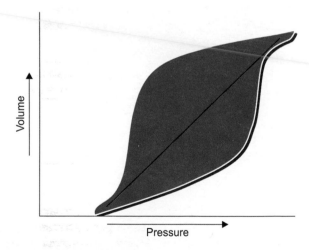

a. Describe the above loop.
b. What is your diagnosis?
c. What is the cause?

Q4.

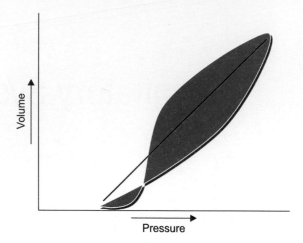

a. Describe above PV loop.
b. What is the commonest cause?

Q5.

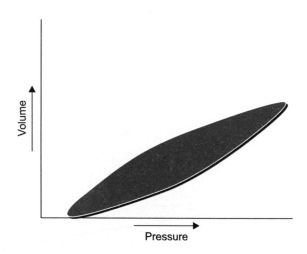

a. Describe the above PV loop.
b. What do you suspect?
c. Enlist 3 causes.

Q6.

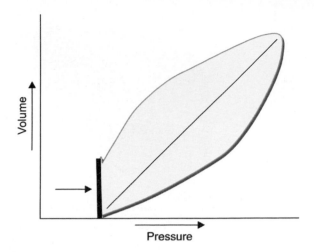

a. Describe the above changes.
b. What do you suspect?
c. Enlist 3 causes.

Q7.

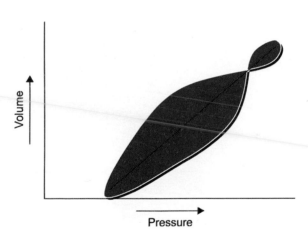

a. Mention what do you suspect in above PV graph.

Q8.

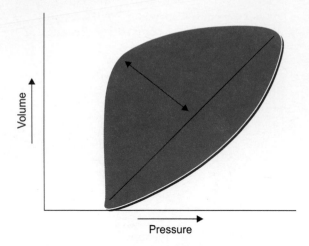

a. Describes the changes of above graph.
b. What pathology can be associated with above changes?
c. Mention 3 common cause of above pathology.

Q9.

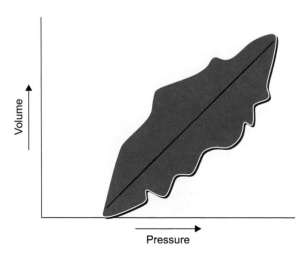

a. Describe above PV loop.
b. Enlist 2 causes.

Q10. Following are representatives of flow-volume curve, here by convention, flow is represented on the Y-axis, volume on the X-axis, expiration as an upward deflection and inspiration as a downward deflection. Name the flow volume curves.

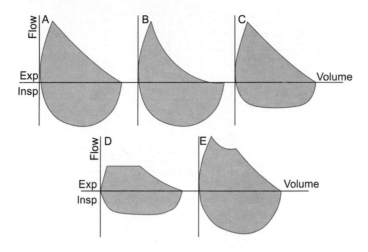

Q11. Following are constructed from spirometric data, please use them to locate the site of air way obstruction.

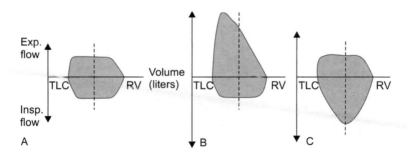

Q12. Intranasal mass

Match the following- can choose more than 1 option

a. Polyp	a. Always intranasal never extranasal
b. Encephalocoele	b. Pulsatile
c. Glioma	c. Trans-illuminable
d. Dermoid	d. Always defect in skull
	e. None of the above

Q13. A 6-week-old infant is presented with on/off history of noisy breathing; on examination you diagnose it as stridor. Baby is otherwise stable with no other clinical concern.

a. What is most likely diagnosis?

b. How do you confirm the diagnosis from history or examination?

c. Enlist 3 causes each of
  i. Persistent causes of stridor
  ii. Acute cause of stridor.

Q14.

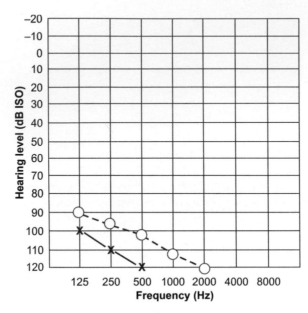

a. What is the audiometric abnormality?
b. Define
  Mild hearing loss
  Moderate hearing loss
  Severe hearing loss
  Profound hearing loss.

Q15. Attached is the audiogram of a 3 year old

a. What is the audiometric abnormality?
b. Enlist 3 common reasons leading in to above abnormality?

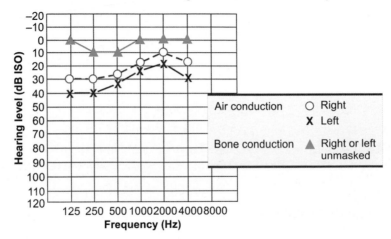

Q16. Answer the following questions.

a. Name the clinical signs which are recommended for assessment of a case of suspected respiratory tract infection under ARI program.

b. A working family has been using a servant maid to care for their 8-month-old child while they go for work. The maid is diagnosed with smear positive pulmonary tuberculosis. PPD test of the 8-month-old is negative. What will you do for this baby?

Q17. Study this arterial blood gas report of a 4-year-old child in the PICU with feeble peripheral pulses.

pH	:	7.28
$PaCO_2$	:	32 mm Hg
PaO_2	:	87 mm Hg
HCO_3	:	12 mMol/L
Base excess	:	8 mMol/L

a. Give the complete ABG diagnosis and possible cause of the abnormality.

b. Name the most appropriate corrective measure for this child.

c. Calculate the predicted carbon dioxide level for this level of bicarbonate.

Q18. Study the arterial blood gas report and answer the questions.

pH	:	7.343
$PaCO_2$	:	60
PaO_2	:	47.8 mm Hg
Bicarbonate	:	32 mMol/L

a. Interpret this blood gas.

b. What is the normal PaO_2 level expected if a child is breathing at room air with normal lungs?

c. Above mentioned ABG was taken when patient was inspiring 60% FiO_2. Calculate the $AaDO_2$ assuming R as 1.

Q19. A baby is admitted to the NICU with persistent pulmonary hypertension (PPHN). He is on ventilator with FiO_2 100%, PIP 35 cm H_2O, PEEP 6 cm H_2O, MAP 14 cm H_2O and SpO_2 85% and he has following loboratory values.

Arterial blood gas (UAC)

pH	:	7.22
$PaCO_2$	:	50 mm Hg
PaO_2	:	50 mm Hg
HCO_3^-	:	14 mMol/L
Na^+	:	136 mEq/L
K^+	:	4 mEq/L
Cl^-	:	103 mEq/L

a. What is the interpretation of this ABG?

b. Calculate oxygenation index.

c. What are the indications for extracorporeal membrane oxygenation (ECMO) in terms of:

  i. $AaDO_2$

  ii. Oxygenation index (OI).

Q20. Answer the following questions.

a. What are the differences between safe and unsafe CSOM? Give three differences.
b. How would you treat safe and unsafe CSOM?

Q21. Study the arterial blood gas report and answer the questions.

pH	:	7.56
$PaCO_2$	:	23.7 mm Hg
PaO_2	:	157 mm Hg
HCO_3	:	24 mMol/L

a. What is your diagnosis?
b. If the baby's Hb is 10 g/dL and SpO_2 is 100%, calculate CaO_2 of the blood.
c. Name one change in ventilator setting that will normalize the blood gas.

Q22. Study the arterial blood gas report of a 12 day old neonate on ventilator and answer the questions.

pH	:	7.30
$PaCO_2$	:	55 mm Hg
PaO_2	:	85 mm Hg
HCO_3	:	31 mMol/L
BE	:	+6.7

a. Interpret this blood gas.
b. What change in bicarbonate you expect if there is rise in $PaCO_2$ by 10 mm (process is chronic)?
c. What change in bicarbonate you expect if there is rise in $PaCO_2$ by 10 mm (process is acute)?

Q23. A 2-year-old male child is brought to a health care centre with findings of a respiratory rate of 60/min without any chest indrawing.

a. Classify the severity of the disease according to IMNCI.
b. What is the choice of antibiotics?

Q24. A 35 week gestation newborn with a birth weight of 2 kg presented with episodes of coughing, cyanosis and respiratory distress specially after feeding at 12 hours of age. Clinically, the neonate was tachypneic, with subcostal and intercostal retractions. The abdomen was scaphoid and there was difficulty in passing a nasogastric tube.

a. What is the diagnosis?
b. Which associated anomalies should be looked for?

Q25. A 6-year-old child after suffering from acute episodes of asthma suddenly started complaining of stabbing pains in the chest radiating to neck. On examination, there was decreased cardiac dullness to percussion and a "mediastinal crunch" was heard on auscultation.

a. Identify the complication.
b. Name two conditions that can give rise to this complication.

Q26. A child with pneumonia on ventilator has following ABG report.

pH	:	7.29
PCO_2	:	60 mm Hg
PaO_2	:	68 mm Hg
HCO_3^-	:	30 mMol/L
SpO_2	:	92%

a. What is the acid base disorder?
b. Is it a simple disorder or mixed?
c. Is it a compensated disorder?
d. What is most likely intervention that will correct the abnormality?

Q27. A 8-year-old boy presented with breathlessness on lying supine. He is markedly pale with liver 4 cm, spleen 5 cm below costal margin and axillary nodes bilaterally 1 × 1 cm.

Answer the following questions after seeing the given chest X-ray
a. What are your findings on this chest X-ray?
b. What is your likely diagnosis based on chest X-ray and clinical findings?
c. How would you confirm?

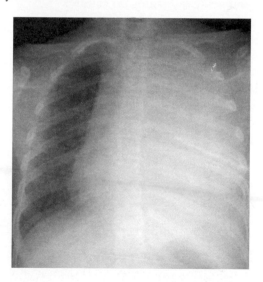

Q28. A 13-year-old girl weighing 26 kg presents with prolonged fever, loss of weight of 6 weeks duration. Her chest X-ray is shown below.

a. List the findings.
b. She was investigated and had PPD 18 × 18 mm. GA for AFB were negative. The treating pediatrician decided to start ATT in this patient. Give the following information:
    i. Category of the disease (WHO-RNTP).
    ii. Drug combination and duration.

c. At the end of treatment, the patient is afebrile, asymptomatic and weighs 33 kg. Her repeat chest X-ray shows 20% residual disease. The repeat PPD ordered by the doctor is 20 × 20 mm.
   i. What is the relevance of the increase in the PPD?
   ii. What is the optimal future course?

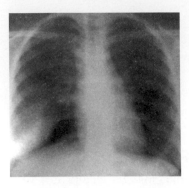

Q29. Answer the following questions on asthma.

a. What is the grade of asthma severity in a child having?
   - Symptoms of airflow obstruction > once a day.
   - Night time symptoms > once a week.
   - PEF—60–80% of personal best with > 30% of diurnal variation.
b. What would be the pulmonary score/severity of asthma exacerbation in a 7 year old child with a respiratory rate of 35, terminal expiratory wheeze and mild increase in work of breathing?

Q30. Answer the following questions.

a. Name the following device.

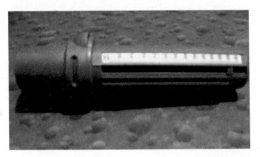

b. What would be the approximate normal value of PEFR of a subject standing 120 cm tall?
c. What does spirometer measures?

Q31. Answer the following questions on pneumonia.

a. Resistance to penicillin in streptococcal pneumonia is mediated by_____.
b. The most important indirect marker of PCP *(P. carinii)* pneumonia is _.
c. Chest radiograph findings typical of PCP pneumonia is _____.

Q 32. A 4-year-old girl presents with fever and a cough. She had developed a temperature at the day care center earlier in the day and her mother was asked to collect her. On arrival in the emergency department she looks toxic, has a temperature of 39.8°C and a slight cough. Mother reports she is refusing fluids. On examination she is sitting on mother's knees quietly, she looks flushed and anxious. You notice a soft inspiratory stridor, tracheal tug and intercostal recessions. Her respiratory rate is 40 breaths per minute and heart rate 140 beats per min. Arterial oxygen saturations are 92% in room air.

a. What is your most likely diagnosis?
b. What characteristic posture does a child usually adopt to find some relief in such a case?
c. How do you confirm the diagnosis in this case and what precautions will you take?
d. What characteristic sign is seen on X-ray?
e. What immediate management is warranted if such a child collapses suddenly?

Q 33. During the winter season a 7-month-old child is referred to the emergency department with worsening cough. He was born at term and has been well and thriving up until now. On examination his temperature is 37.6°C. Respiratory rate 70 bpm, heart rate 130 bpm. He has moderate intercostal recessions and his arterial oxygen saturations are 88% on room air. Auscultation of his chest reveals bilateral scattered fine crepts.

a. What is your likely diagnosis?
b. What is the main causative organism for this ? Give 2 other causative organisms.
c. What is the mainstay of treatment?
d. Which babies are prone to this disease and how do you prevent disease in them?

Q 34. A 7-month-old boy is referred to the pediatric emergency department in January with a fever of 38.1°C and a cough. He also has had diarrhoea on and off for three months. His birth weight at term was plotted on the 75th centile and has dropped to the 25th centile. Mother reports that he usually has a very good appetite but has taken only 75% of feeds over the last three days. On clinical examination you find a respiratory rate of 50 bpm, mild intercostal recessions and bilateral crepitations. Abdominal examination is unremarkable.

a. What is your likely diagnosis?
b. Mention 3 other respiratory manifestations of this disease.
c. Mention 2 endocrine manifestations of this disease.
d. Give common organisms that colonise the airways in this disease.
e. What is the standard diagnostic test for this condition?

Q 35. A 12-year-old patient with homozygous sickle-cell disease presents to the emergency department during the winter months with a fever of

39.5°C and increasing pain in both legs over the last 6 hours. Over the last hour he has complained of right-sided chest pain. Further examination reveals a respiratory rate of 44 breaths per min and a heart rate of 140 beats per min. His arterial oxygen saturation is 85% in air.

a. What is your most likely diagnosis?
b. What do you expect in chest X-ray of this patient?
c. What is the most common preceding event for this condition?
d. Give 2 ways that help to reduce the frequency of such episodes.

Q 36. A 5-month-old infant presents to the emergency department with paroxysms of coughing. She has had one episode of going blue while feeding and coughing that morning. She has not received her routine immunizations, as mother has been concerned with all the problems of MMR, so has not given any vaccines. You decide to admit the child to the ward for further observation.

a. What possibility do you suspect in this baby?
b. What two most relevant investigations will you send?
c. The child was discharged from the ward 4 days later. She was reviewed in clinic 4 weeks after discharge. Her mother is very concerned that she is still coughing. How do you convince the mother?
d. What complications are expected in untreated cases?

Q 37. A 6-year-old boy is seen in the emergency department with breathlessness and fever. His mother reports that he had a cough and fever 10 days ago, which settled with supportive treatment alone. He had developed a high fever again over the last 12 hours and become increasingly breathless. He has a slight cough, is tachypneic and complains of right-sided chest pain. He requires 5 L of facemask oxygen to maintain arterial oxygen saturations at 94%. On clinical examination of the chest there is reduced expansion on the right, dullness on percussion of the right lower zone and no audible air entry over this area.

a. What is your most likely diagnosis?
b. Pleural effusion is said to be purulent when leukocytes are ————
c. Give 4 diagnostic features on pleural fluid examination to call it as empyema.

Q 38. A 28-month-old child presents to ER with fever of 102°F and a cough. Physical examination reveals right sided rales and a chest X-ray confirms a right middle lobe infiltrate. You note that the patient has been seen twice in last month with diagnosis of RML infiltrates both confirmed by chest X-ray. This child is otherwise healthy with no medical concerns. A Mantoux test was done which was negative.

a. What is the most likely diagnosis causing this "secondary pneumonia"?
b. What other presentations could a child with this diagnosis have?
c. What bronchus is most likely to be affected?
d. How do you make the diagnosis and how do you confirm it?
e. What is the most common age of presentation for this?

Q 39. Answer the following questions on ventilation.

a. A child is getting ventilated by "pressure limited' ventilator whose ABG shows $PaCO_2$ value of 70 mm Hg with normal oxygenation. Which of the following is the best change in the ventilator settings to achieve normocapnea?

b. A patient is breathing spontaneously on a ventilator, which delivers a pressure of 5 cm of H_2O throughout his respiration. What is this mode of ventilation called?

c. What is the expiratory time in a ventilatory setting of pressure control ventilation with I : E ratio of 1 : 2 with 10% pause at the rate of 20 breaths per minute?

d. In a volume flow curve, a child of age 4 years is intubated with an ET tube of 4 mm size. The inspiratory tidal volume is 12 ml but expiratory tidal volume is only 4 ml. What does this indicate?

e. What should be the ventilator strategy in a child with acute severe asthma?

Q 40. A newborn infant is in respiratory distress and requires several attempts at resuscitation in the delivery room because of difficulty in breathing and frequent cyanosis. The neonatologist notes that during crying, her breathing improves and breath and heart sounds are normal. Direct laryngoscopy is unremarkable as well. Deep inspirations by the neonate are ineffective.

a. What is your likely diagnosis?

b. What will be your immediate and most effective intervention?

c. Give 2 conditions commonly associated with this entity.

Q 41. A 4-year-old child complains of ear pain. He has a temperature of 102.1°F (38.9°C) and has had a cold for several days, but he has been eating well and his activity has been essentially normal.

a. What is the most likely diagnosis?

b. What is the best therapy?

c. What is the most common causative organism for this?

ANSWERS

A 1:

Right middle lobe
Lateral and medial bronchus—lying supine with the body a quarter turned to the left maintained by a pillow under the right side from shoulder to hip and foot end raised by 14 inches (35 cm).

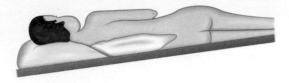

Lingula Left
Superior and inferior bronchus—lying supine with the body a quarter turned the right maintained by a pillow under the left side from shoulder to hip and foot end raised by 14 inches (35 cm).

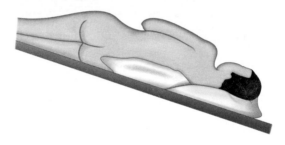

A 2:

Disorder	
a. Metabolic acidosis	$(P_{CO2}) = 1.5 \times (HCO_3^-) + 8 \pm 2$
b. Metabolic alkalosis	(P_{CO2}) increase by 7_{mmHg} for each 10 mEq/L increase in (HCO_3^-)

A 3:
a. PV loop shows bird beak at the top of the loop
b. Overdistension
c. VT Set too high (press vent).

A 4:
a. Figure of eight expiration or A pig tail at the bottom. The bigger the pig tail, the higher the patient WOB to trigger the breath
b Increase work of breathing, Trigger set is too high.

A 5:

a. There is slow rising inspiratory limb. Change in volume is little as compared to change in pressure that is dynamic compliance is less
b. Decreased Lung compliance
c. RDS, ARDS, Pneumothorax, Abdominal distension.

A 6:

a. Pressure-Volume loop fails to close, Tidal volume waveform dose not reach baseline at end-expiration
b. Air Leak
c. ET Leak, Small size, wrong placement, tubing detached, water seal detached, sensor not in place.

A 7:

a. Low minute volume, Inadequate flow, trigger set to high, little separation between inflation and deflation limbs of PV loop.

A 8:

a. Increased expiratory resistive work
b. Obstructive air way diseases
c. Meconium aspiration syndrome
   Bronchopulmonary dysplesia

A 9:

a. Noisy signals on both loops
b. Turbulence due to
   i. Water in circuit
   ii. Airway Secretions.

A 10:

a. NORMAL
b. Intrathoracic peripheral airway obstruction
c. Variable extrathoracic airway obstruction
d. Fixed airway obstruction
e. Variable extrathoracic central airway obstruction.

A 11:

a. Fixed obstruction intra or extra thoracic
b. Extrathoracic obstruction (variable)
c. Intra thoracic obstruction (variable)

A 12:

a. A
b. BCD
c. E
d. E.

A 13:

a. Laryngomalacia
b. Stridor disappears when the child lies prone

Persistent causes of stridor	Acute cause of stridor
Laryngomalacia	Acute laryngotracheobronchitis
Subglottic stenosis	Acute epiglottitis
Vocal cord palsy	Foreign body or inhaled hot gas
Vascular ring	Acute angioneurotic oedema
Laryngeal Web/cleft	Diphtheria
Cysts of the posterior tongue	Expanding mediastinal mass
Cysts of the aryepiglottic folds.	

A 14:

a. Bilateral Profound hearing loss
b.
Mild	25–35 Db
Moderate	40–60 Db
Severe	60–90 Db
Profound	> 90 Db.

A 15:

a. A .Bilateral conductive hearing loss
b.

- Cerumen (earwax)
- Otitis externa (ear infection
- Acute otitis media
- Serous otitis media.

A 16:

a.   i. Tachypnea
     ii. Retractions
    iii. Central cyanosis
     iv. Grunting.
      v. Fever.
b. For infants, if the mother or any other household member is smear positive, then INH chemoprophylaxis @ 5 mg/kg is given for 3 months, followed by a Mantoux test. If Mantoux test is negative (< 6 mm induration) then stop chemoprophylaxis and give BCG, if not given previously. If Mantoux test is positive (≥ 6 mm induration) then continue chemoprophylaxis for 3 more months (total duration of 6 months).

A 17:

a. Uncompensated metabolic acidosis; shock
b. Fluid bolus
c. $12 \times 1.5 + 8 \pm 2 = 24\text{–}28$ mm Hg.

A 18:

a. Uncompensated respiratory acidosis
b. 80–100 mm Hg.

c. $AaDO_2$ $= PAO_2 - PaO_2$
PAO_2 $= (760-47) FiO_2 - PCO_2/RQ$
$= 713 \times 0.6-60 = 367.8$
So $AaDO_2$ $= 367.8 - 47.8 = 320.$

A 19:

a. Mixed acidosis with hypoxemia.

b. $OI = \dfrac{MAP \times FiO_2}{Postductal\ PO_2} \times 100 = \dfrac{14 \times 1}{50} \times 100 = 28$

c. i. Oxygen gradient > 600 mm Hg for 12 hour or > 610 mm Hg at 8 hour or 605 mm Hg for 4 hours
   ii. OI > 40.

A 20:

a. Safe—tubotympanic disease, residual of ASOM, central perforation, copious discharge, granulation absent, conductive loss, sclerotic changes on X-ray
   Unsafe—atticoantral, perforation in attic, granulation common, cholesteatoma formed with destruction of mastoid bone, scanty discharge, mixed hearing loss

b. Tympanoplasty (safe), mastoidectomy (unsafe).

A 21:

a. Respiratory alkalosis.
b. CaO_2: Hb% (10) × 1.34 mL × 100/(100 + 0.003 × 157) = 14.77 mL.
c. Decrease PIP.

A 22:

a. Respiratory acidosis with partial metabolic compensation
b. 3.5 mmol/L; HCO_3 increases by 3.5 for each 10 mm Hg rise in PCO_2
c. 1 mmol/L; HCO_3 increases by 1 for each 10 mm Hg rise in PCO_2.

A 23:

a. Pneumonia
b. Amoxycillin and septran.

A 24:

a. Esophageal atresia
b. Vater/vactrel.

A 25:

a. Pneumomediastinum
b. Trauma, dental extraction, esophageal perforation.

A 26:

a. Respiratory acidosis
b. Simple
c. Uncompensated

d. Increase ventilator rate
Decrease tube length
Clear tube of secretions, if present.

A 27:

a. Left sided opacity with trachea shifted to right with chest tube in situ on left
b. Mediastinal mass with left sided pleural effusion cause? Lymphoma T cell
c. Bone marrow
Pleural fluid analysis for immunophenotyping and malignant cells.

A 28:

a. Paratracheal LN and right hilar LN.
b.   i. Category 3
   ii. 2 RHZ/4 RH.
c.   i. No relevance in clinical decisions in this case now
   ii. No further treatment. Only follow up required now.

A 29:

a. Moderate persistent.
b. 3 (mild).

A 30:

a. Peak flow meter
b. 200 liters/min
Formula for approximate normal PEFR for a given height:
PEFR (L/min) = [ht. (in cm) – 80] × 5.
c. Vital capacity and its subdivisions and expiratory (or inspiratory) flow rate.

A 31:

a. Penicillin binding proteins with altered affinity for penicillin
b. Hypoxemia (i.e., PaO_2 < 80 mm Hg in room air)
c. Interstitial infiltrates beginning in the perihilar region and spreading to the periphery. Apices spared until later in the disease.

A 32:

a. Acute epiglottitis.
b. Tripod position—sitting upright and leaning forwards with chin up and mouth open while bracing on the arms.
c. Direct visualization of large, 'cherry red' swollen epiglottis. Ensure availability of resuscitation or tracheostomy equipments.
d. Lateral neck X-ray shows 'thumb sign'.
e. Establishing an airway by nasotracheal intubation or less often by tracheostomy, regardless of the degree of apparent respiratory distress.

A 33:

a. Acute bronchiolitis.
b. RSV is responsible for > 50% cases. Other viruses include parainfluenza, adenovirus, mycoplasma and human meta pneumovirus.

c. Cool humidified oxygen to prevent hypoxemia.

d. Premature babies, CLD, congenital heart disease, immunodeficient babies.

Administration of pooled hyperimmune RSV IVIG; and Palivizumab, intramuscular monoclonal antibody to RSV F protein before and during RSV season in infants < 2 years.

A 34:

a. Cystic fibrosis. The presenting history might at first suggest bronchiolitis (age, season, clinical presentation but the weight loss is out of proportion with the short history of reduced feeds). Ongoing diarrhea, weight loss and chest signs/symptoms should alert you to a possible diagnosis of cystic fibrosis.

b. Bronchiectasis, sinusitis, nasal polyps, hemoptysis, pneumothorax, cor pulmonale, mucoid impaction of bronchi.

c. Delayed puberty, infertility, diabetes mellitus, gynecomastia.

d. *Staph aureus, Pseudomonas aeruginosa, Burkholderia cepacia.*

e. Quantitative sweat test using pilocarpine electrophoresis ($Cl^- \leq 60\,mEq/L$) in conjunction with 1 or more of the following: typical chronic obstructive pulmonary disease, documented exocrine pancreatic insufficiency or a positive family history.

A 35:

a. Acute chest syndrome.

b. Radiographs may show single lobe involvement, most often left lower lobe, and when multiple lobes are involved, usually both lower lobes are affected. New radiodensities appear during each episode.

c. Painful episodes requiring opioids.

d. Incentive spirometry, avoidance of overhydration, early ambulation in patients admitted with vaso-occlusive crisis.

A 36:

a. Pertussis.

b. Full blood count to look for absolute lymphocytosis and pernasal swab for direct fluorescent antibody testing for pertussis.

c. Whooping cough (pertussis) is a respiratory tract infection characterized by paroxysms of coughing followed by a 'whoop' (sudden massive inspiratory effort with a narrowed glottis). It is caused by the bacterium *Bordetella pertussis,* which has an incubation period of 7 to 10 days usually, but this can occasionally be as long as 21 days. Cough episodes in pertussis is slow to resolve even after adequate antibiotic treatment.

d. Pre-term infants and those with underlying cardiac, pulmonary or neuromuscular problems are at high risk of complications of pertussis. These include pneumonia, seizures, encephalopathy and death.

A 37:

a. Right pleural effusion.

b. >5000/mm^3.

c. • Purulent appearance

- Cell count >5000; cell type PMN
- Pleural fluid/serum LDH > 0.6
- Pleural fluid/serum protein > 0.5
- Pleural fluid LDH > 1000 U/L
- Pleural fluid glucose very low (<40 mg/dL)
- 85% positive for gram stain unless patient received prior antibiotics.

A 38:

a. Foreign body aspiration.
b. Respiratory distress, choking, lung collapse, hyperinflation on one side (ball valve mechanism).
c. Right main bronchus.
d. Bronchoscopy.
e. 1–3 years.

A 39:

a. Increase rate, decrease tube size, clear obstructed tube.
b. CPAP.
c. 2 seconds.
d. Peritubal leak.
e. Low PEEP with long expiratory time.

A 40:

a. Choanal atresia.
b. Inserting an oropharyngeal airway.
c. CHARGE syndrome
   *C*oloboma.
   *H*eart disease
   *A*tresia choanae
   *R*etarded growth and development or CNS anomalies or both
   *G*enital anomalies or hypogonadism or both
   *E*ar anomalies or deafness or both.

A 41:

a. Acute otitis media.
b. Oral antibiotics (Amoxicillin at higher dose of 80–100 mg/kg/day for 10 days).
c. *Streptococcus pneumoniae* followed by *H. influenzae.*

Statistics

QUESTIONS

Q1. Answer the following.

a. Define median, 1st quartile and 3rd quartile.
b. What is the difference between rate and ratio?
c. What is the basic difference between a 'case control' and 'cohort' study design?
d. What is the difference between incidence and prevalence?

Q2. Interpret the following statement.

In a RCT, the 'odds' of developing HMD were 0.55 (95% CI 0.3–2.1) in infants whose mothers were given 'antenatal steroids'.

Q3. In a small government hospital, 60% of early neonatal deaths have low-birth-weight. It is also seen that nearly 5% births in this hospital die within a week and about 30% births have low-birth-weight. Calculate the probability that a low-birth-weight baby would die in early neonatal period.

Q4. The height of 10 children of the same age group is given: (all in cm).

101, 98, 98, 99, 102, 101,100, 98, 101, 101

Calculate:
a. Mean
b. Mode
c. Median.

Q5. At a camp, a new model of mass miniature radiography was used to screen for tuberculosis. Subsequently, the subjects were also subjected to CT scan of the chest to confirm whether the results were reliable or not. The results were as follows.

Screening test	Diseased	Not diseased
Positive	a (TP)	b (FP)
Negative	c (FN)	d (TN)

Calculate (give formulae)
a. Specificity
b. Sensitivity
c. Positive predictive value
d. Negative predictive value.

Q6. Out of 50 babies delivered in a hospital, 10 were stillbirths. Out of this, 5 were less than 1000 g. Out of the survivors, 5 died in first month of life.
a. Calculate:
   1. Stillbirth rate.
   2. Neonatal mortality rate.
b. Define perinatal mortality rate.

Q7. Out of a population of 5000 children in a village, 500 cases of malnutrition already exist. There are 100 newly diagnosed cases in a year. 20 children died of malnutrition. Calculate.
a. Prevalence rate.
b. Incidence rate.
c. Case fatality rate.
d. What is advantage of calculating prevalence rate?

Q8. Answer the following questions.
a. Define p-value.
b. In a study of 30 patients of liver cirrhosis, enzyme level was evaluated before and after treatment. What statistical test would you apply in this case?
c. When do you apply non-parametric test?

Q9.
a. Calculate the odd's ratio in the given case control study design:

Exposure (risk factor)	Disease present	Disease absent
Yes	a	b
No	c	d
Total	a + c	b + d

b. What is the significance of the term odds ratio in statistical terms?

Q10.

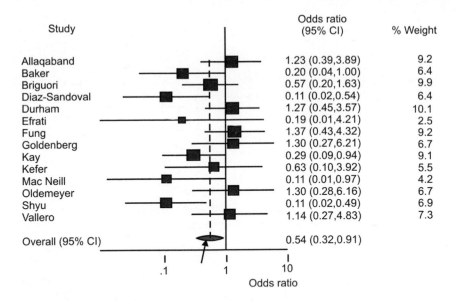

Study	Odds ratio (95% CI)	% Weight
Allaqaband	1.23 (0.39,3.89)	9.2
Baker	0.20 (0.04,1.00)	6.4
Briguori	0.57 (0.20,1.63)	9.9
Diaz-Sandoval	0.11 (0.02,0.54)	6.4
Durham	1.27 (0.45,3.57)	10.1
Efrati	0.19 (0.01,4.21)	2.5
Fung	1.37 (0.43,4.32)	9.2
Goldenberg	1.30 (0.27,6.21)	6.7
Kay	0.29 (0.09,0.94)	9.1
Kefer	0.63 (0.10,3.92)	5.5
Mac Neill	0.11 (0.01,0.97)	4.2
Oldemeyer	1.30 (0.28,6.16)	6.7
Shyu	0.11 (0.02,0.49)	6.9
Vallero	1.14 (0.27,4.83)	7.3
Overall (95% CI)	0.54 (0.32,0.91)	

a. What is this plot known as? And where are they primarily used?
b. What is the arrowed figure known as?
c. In this plot which study has the best association regarding the outcome?

Q11. You are doing a study "Is zinc better than racecadotril for diarrhea" and the results are like this.

Zinc		Racecadotril	
Improvement	Nil	Improvement	Nil
12	27	6	20

a. Calculate the relative risk.
b. What does it signify?

Q12.
a. In an area the under 5 mortality is 5/1000 live births. Calculate the child survival index in that area.
b. What is the appropriate statistical test to compare two means?
c. What is the appropriate statistical test to compare two proportions?

Q13.

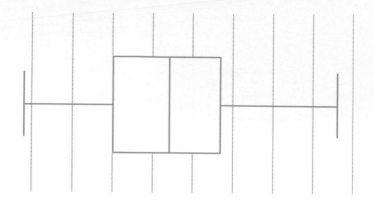

a. What is this plot known as?
b. What is this used for?
c. Describe the plot.

Q14. In an international clinical trial, two chemotherapy treatments are being compared (Choose the correct answer for each of the following questions).

a. How are systematic differences between treatment groups best minimized?
    i. Analyze results by country separately.
    ii. Multivariate analysis.
    iii. Patient stratification.
    iv. Prognostic factor analysis.
    v. Randomization.

b. What is the rationale for conducting a clinical trial in a double blind manner?
    i. It effectively increases the size of the trial by using each patient as their own control.
    ii. It increases comparability of patient characteristics in the treatment and control groups.
    iii. It increases the precision of the estimated effect.
    iv. It reduces systematic bias between the treatment and the control groups.
    v. It reduces the effects of sampling variations.

c. In a normal distribution the mean of the data will be similar to the:
    i. Maximum.
    ii. Median.
    iii. Range.
    iv. Standard deviation.
    v. Standard error.

d. The table below shows the number of adverse effects reported in a randomized trial comparing two treatments—A and B.

Treatment group		Adverse events	
	Yes	No	Total
A	4	28	32
B	16	12	28
Total	20	40	60

The odds ratio of having an adverse event in group A is:
  i. 4/16
 ii. 4/20
iii. 4/28
 iv. 4/32
  v. 4/60

Q15. Calculate sensitivity, specificity, positive and negative predictive value of ECG test for myocardial infarction (MI) from the data given below.

ECG	M I		Total
	Present	Absent	
Positive	300	100	400
Negative	25	75	100
Total	325	175	500

Q16. Consider the following reterospective data on the parity of mothers of 210 normal and 140 IUGR babies.

IUGR	Parity < 3	Parity > 3	Total
Present	98	112	210
Absent	92	48	140

a. What are the odds for mothers with parity < 3 giving birth to IUGR baby as compared to mother with parity > 3?
b. What is the difference between odds ratio and relative risk?

Q17. Which of the following statements are true regarding power of a study?

a. Power is the probability of rightly rejecting a null hypothesis when it is false.
b. Power is directly related to the magnitude of the difference to be detected.
c. Power increases as the sample size increases.
d. An increase in the level of significance is a negative feature whereas an increase in power is a positive feature of a statistical test. These should be balanced.
e. Power increases if a higher probability of type I error can be tolerated.

Q18. State true/false regarding case control study design.

a. A case control study is done to generate a hypothesis.
b. A case control study requires a large number of subjects and large number of controls.
c. A case control study cannot be retrospective.
d. A case control study is an analytical study.
e. A case control study is an observational study.

Q19. Match the items with appropriate scale of measurement.

a. Number of cigarettes smoked   i.   Ordinal
b. Body temperature   ii. Ratio
c. Age in completed years   iii. Interval
d. Age in categories, e.g. child,   iv. Metric
   adolescent, adult
e. Stage of a cancer   v.   Continous variable
f. Blood sugar levels   vi. Discrete variable

Q20.

a. You use a histological test for cancer that has sensitivity, specificity, positive predictivity and negative predictivity in excess of 90%. Which of the four indicators would you use to reassure a patient that the positive test could still be an error?
b. Which test would you use for ruling out a disease in a patient?
c. Which test would you use for confirming a disease in a patient?

Q21. Consider the following data.

- Total population of children in an area   -   1300
- Protected against measles by vaccination   -   800
- Total cases of measles in one year   -   10
- Primary cases   -   2
- Number of susceptible children coming in contact   -   15
  of primary cases
- Secondary cases that received infection from primary   -   8
  cases within the infective period

a. Calculate attack rate of measles.
b. Calculate secondary attack rate of measles.

Q22. In a hospital data, fetal deaths during the late gestation period ($\geq$ 28 weeks) was found to be only 2%. Out of all the remaining live births, 3% died within 1 week. What is the perinatal mortality rate in this hospital?

ANSWERS

A 1:

a. If the observations are arranged in ascending or descending order:
Median: 50% observations are below and 50% are above this value.
1st Quartile: 25% observations are below and 75% are above this value.
3rd Quartile: 75% observations are below and 25% are above this value.

b. *Rate:* Numerator is part of denominator
Ratio: Numerator is not part of denominator.

c. Case control study is retrospective and cohort study is prospective.

d. *Incidence:* The number of new cases occurring in defined population during a specified period of time.
Prevalence: Number of all cases old and new at a given point of time or over a period of time in a given population.

A 2:

In infants of mothers who had received antenatal steroids the chances of developing HMD are 45% less as compared to those whose mother had not received antenatal steroids. However, the 95% confidence intervals are not significant.

A 3: 10%

Hint – Apply Bayes' rule : $P(\text{disease/complaint}) = \dfrac{P(\text{complaint/disease}) \times P(\text{disease})}{P(\text{complaint})}$

P (LBW/early neonatal death) = 0.60

P (early neonatal death) = 0.05   and   P (LBW) = 0.30

$P(\text{early neonatal death/LBW}) = \dfrac{P(\text{LBW/early neonatal death}) \times P(\text{early neonatal death})}{\times P(\text{LBW})}$

$= \dfrac{0.60 \times 0.05}{0.30} = 0.10 = 10\%$

A 4: First arrange all values in ascending or descending order

98, 98, 98, 99, 100, 101, 101, 101, 101, 102

a. Mean = Sum of all/total no = 1000/10 = 100

b. Median = Middle value in ascending or descending order
(100 + 101)/2 = 100.5

c. Mode = That value which is the most frequent
(comes for most times) = 101

A 5:

a. Specificity = True negative = $d/(b + d) \times 100$

b. Sensitivity = True positive = $a/(a + c) \times 100$

c. Positive predictive value = True positive/all positive =
$$a/(a + b) \times 100$$

d. Negative predictive value = True negative/All negatives =
$$d/(c + d) \times 100$$

A 6:

a.

1. Stillbirth rate = $\dfrac{\text{No of fetal deaths (with weight > 1000 g)}}{\text{Total live + stillbirths (with weight > 1000 g)}} \times 1000$

$$\frac{5}{40 + 5} \times 1000 = \frac{1000}{9} = 111.1$$

2. Neonatal mortality rate = $\dfrac{\text{No of deaths in first month}}{\text{Total live births}} \times 1000$

$$\frac{5}{40} \times 1000 = 125$$

b. Perinatal mortality rate is total number of late fetal deaths (> 28 weeks of gestation or fetus > 1000 grams) +

$$\frac{\text{neonatal deaths in the first seven days of life}}{\text{total live births}}$$

A 7:

a. Prevalence rate:

$$\frac{\text{No of existing + new cases}}{\text{Population at risk}} \times 100 = \frac{(500 + 100) \times 100}{5000} = \frac{600 \times 100}{5000} = 12$$

b. Incidence rate:

$$\frac{\begin{array}{c}\text{No of new cases of specific disease}\\ \text{during a given period of time}\end{array}}{\text{Population at risk}} \times 1000 = \frac{100 \times 1000}{5000} = 20$$

c. Case fatality rate:

$$\frac{\text{Total no of deaths due to a particular disease}}{\text{Total no of cases due to the same disease}} \times 100 = \frac{20}{(500 + 100)} \times 100$$

$$= \frac{20 \times 100}{600} = 3.33$$

d. Advantage:
    i. To estimate magnitude of health disease problem in country.
    ii. To identify potential risk population.
    iii. For administrative and planning purposes.

A 8:

a. It is the probability of type 1 error, i.e. the chance that a difference or association is concluded when actually there is none.
b. Paired 't' test.
c. Non-parametric test is applied when distribution is non-Gaussian and sample size is small.

A 9:

a. For case control studies, ratio of odds

$$= \frac{a/c}{b/d} = ad/bc$$

b. Odds ratio is a measure of strength of association between outcome and antecedent
   OR = 1 means that the risk factor has no association with the disease
   OR>1 suggests risk factor associated with increased disease
   OR<1 suggests risk factor protective against disease.

A 10:

a. Forest plot are used in meta-analysis.
b. Diamond.
c. Study done by Kay.

A 11:

a. RR (Treatment) is $= \dfrac{n\,(Exposed)}{n\,(Non\ exposed)}$

$$= \frac{12/39}{6/26} = 1.52$$

b. Outcome variable is 1.52 times more in the zinc group than in the racecadotril group.

A 12.

a. Child survival index $= \dfrac{1000 - \text{under 5 mortality}}{10}$

$$= 1000\text{-}5/10 = 99.5$$

b. Student 't' test
c. Chi-square test

A 13:

a. Box-and-whisker plot.
b. They display a statistical summary of a variables : median, quartiles, range and extreme values.
c. The central box represents the values from the lower to upper quartile (25 to 75 percentile).
The middle line represents the median.
The horizontal line extends from the minimum to the maximum value, excluding *outside* and *far out* values which are displayed as separate points.

A 14:

a. v (Randomisation).
b. iv (Reduces systematic bias between the treatment and control groups).
c. ii (Median).
d. iii (4/28).

A 15:

$$\text{Sensitivity} = 300/325 = 92.3\%$$
$$\text{Specificity} = 75/175 = 42.9\%$$
$$\text{PPV} = 300/400 = 75\%$$
$$\text{NPV} = 75/100 = 75\%$$

A 16:

a. Ods ratio = ad/bc
   = 98 × 48/92 × 112 = 0.45
b. Relative risk is applicable only to prospective studies while odds ratio is used only in retrospective studies.

A 17:

All the given statements are correct.

A 18:

a. False: It tests already set up hypothesis.
b. False: It can be done on relatively small number of cases and controls because status of disease in the subjects is already known.
c. False: It is always retrospective.
d. True: Involves comparison of presence of an antecedent in cases and controls.
e. True: It does not involve any human interventions. Only natural occurrence is observed.

A 19:

a. Number of cigarettes smoked   -   Ratio
b. Body temperature   -   Interval
c. Age in completed years   -   Metric
d. Age in categories, e.g. child,   -   Ordinal
   adolescent, adult
e. Stage of a cancer   -   Discrete variable
f. Blood sugar levels   -   Continous variable

A 20:

a. Positive predictive value is the chance of presence of the disease when the test is positive. If this is 90%, there is still a chance of 10% that the disease is not present. Thus PPV can be used to reassure the patient that there is still some chance of absence of disease despite positive test.
b. Test with high negative predictive value (NPV).
c. Test with high positive predictive value (PPV).

A 21:

a. Attack rate of measles = $\dfrac{\text{No. of cases/spells in a year}}{\text{No. at risk for measles}}$

$$= 10/(1300–800) = 10/500 = 2\%$$

b. Secondary attack rate = $\dfrac{\text{secondary cases}}{\text{No. of susceptible children coming in contact}}$

$$= 8/15 = 53\%$$

A 22: • 49/1000.
- Fetal deaths = 2%
- So live births out of 100 pregnancies ($\geq$ 28 weeks gestation) = 98
- So death within first week = 3% of 98 = 2.94

$$\text{PMR} = \frac{\text{Still birth + death within one week}}{\text{Still birth + live birth}} = \frac{2 + 2.94}{2 + 98}$$

$$= 4.94\% = 49/1000 \text{ (as it is a rate and not ratio)}$$

Miscellaneous

QUESTIONS

Q1. Designing of Pediatric ICU's in India- IAP-Recommendations
a. What is the recommended noise level during daytime?
b. What is the recommended noise level during night time?
c. What is the recommended floor area per patient?
d. What is the recommended minimal distance between two bed center?
e. What is the ideal bed strength for economic viability of each PICU?
f. What is the Ideal and minimal nurse to patient ratio?

Q2.
a. How do you classify dental fracture?
b. A child falls and knocks out his front tooth. How would the treatment differ in a 4 year old and 14 year old?
c. Enlist 3 mediums to transport avulsed tooth.

Q3.

	Site of sample collection	Earliest gestation age to perform the test
CVS or CVB		
Amniocentesis		
Cordocentesis		

Q4. Yes/No
a. In general, do minor have the right to give consent for their own treatment?
b. In an emergency, is it necessary to obtain consent in order to treat a child?
c. Can a child who lives away from home, is no longer subject to parental control, is economically self-supporting

d. Can a child who is sufficiently mature to understand the nature of his/ her illness and the potential risks and benefits of proposed therapy, give or refuse consent to treatment?

e. May Jehovah's witness parents refuse blood transfusion for their minor children?

Q5.

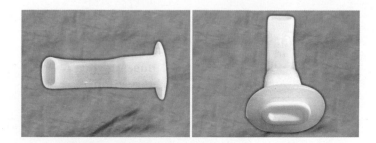

a. What is the device shown?
b. What is the usage of device?
c. How is the correct size measured?
d. How do you insert the device?
e. Enlist 2 complication associated with the usage of the device.

Q6. A 2-year-child presents with the following:

- 5 episodes of abscesses in 6 months
- Photosensitivity
- Photophobia
- Light skin and silvery hair.

Peripheral smear shows large inclusions in all nucleated blood cells.

a. What is the diagnosis?
b. What is the mode of inheritance?
c. What is the neurological manifestation?
d. What is the treatment?

Q7. Select the answers

a. Small (pinhead to 1 cm), pearly papules with translucent tops and waxy, whitish material inside, distributed on the face and anterior trunk. Some lesions are umbilicated.
b. Soft, flesh-colored papular or pedunculated lesions around the genitalia and rectum.
c. Oval, maculopapular lesions oriented with the long axis along skin tension lines.
d. Characteristically pruritic.
   i. Miliaria rubra
   ii. Verrucae vulgaris
   iii. Condyloma acuminatum
   iv. Molluscum contagiosum
   v. Pityriasis rosea.

Q8. Study the photograph shown below and answer the following questions.

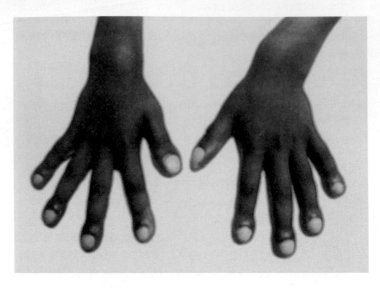

a. Identify the spot with its grade.
b. Give the grading of this condition.

Q9. A 2-month-old girl is admitted with acute viral myocarditis. She is on dopamine, amrinone, ranitidine and cefotaxime. Her platelet count has reduced from 200,000 to 50000/cu mm over past 5 days.

a. This thrombocytopenia is most likely due to:
   i. Ranitidine.
   ii. Amrinone.
   iii. Viral suppression of bone marrow.
   iv. Heparin in her central venous catheter.
   v. Vascular congestion of spleen from right heart failure.
b. On what two factors does the severity of thrombocytopenia depend upon in this case?
c. What class of drug is this?
d. What is the mechanism of action of this drug?

Q10. Give the best possible answer to the following questions.

a. A 7-month-old male baby has just returned from operating room after complete repair of tetralogy of Fallot. Patient is mottled and has cool extremities. He has good chest rise with ventilator breaths. CVP is 6 cm, blood pressure is 64/40 mm Hg and heart rate is 165/min. He is on dobutamine at 10 mic/kg/min and nitroglycerine at 1 mic/kg/min. His Hb is 12 g/dL. Oxygen saturation is 95% on 60% oxygen. Most appropriate first step would be:
   i. Give 10 mL/kg fluid.
   ii. Begin epinephrine at 0.05 mic/kg/min.
   iii. Decrease the nitroglycerine to 0.5 mic/kg/min.

    iv. Increase dobutamine to 20 mic/kg/min.

    v. Hyperventilate the patient.

b. What is the commonest ingredient in mosquito repellants?

    i. Pyrethroids.

    ii. Organochlorines.

    iii. Organophosphorus.

    iv. None of the above.

c. Which of the following is not useful in acute methemoglobinemia?

    i. Oxygen therapy.

    ii. Exchange transfusion.

    iii. Methylene blue.

    iv. Vitamin C.

d. Activated charcoal is effective for all of the following *except:*

    i. Phenobarbitones.

    ii. Hydrocarbons.

    iii. Theophylline.

    iv. Organophosphates.

Q11.

a. A 4-year-old child is brought to ER 15 minutes after he has accidentally ingested around one teaspoon of kerosene oil. Which of the following will you do?

    i. Gastric lavage and start antibiotics + steroids.

    ii. Get an X-ray of chest done immediately.

    iii. Observe the child for at least 6 hours.

    iv. All of the above.

b. When do you order for X-ray chest in this case?

c. What is the role of prophylactic antibiotics in a case of kerosene poisoning?

d. What is the most important complication of this condition?

Q12. Organophosphate poisoning.

a. Organophosphate poisoning is characterized by all of the following except:

    i. Miosis.

    ii. Urinary retention.

    iii. Emesis.

    iv. Lacrimation.

b. Name two antidotes for treatment of this poisoning.

c. What is the mechanism of organophosphate poisoning?

d. Enlist four symptoms of cholinergic excess.

Q13. A 7-year-old child has come to pediatric emergency room with bizarre behavior, vomiting and respiratory distress. On examination, child has lots of oral secretions, HR–60/min, BP–90/62 mm Hg and pupils are small.

a. Which toxicity does this child probably has?

b. Write two most common causes of this.

c. What are the four most important steps in the management of this child?

d. What is the commonest delayed complication?

Q14. A 5-year-old child is caught in a house fire and brought to ER with 60% burns. His weight is around 16 kg.

a. What most likely immediate complication is expected in this case and how will you identify this complication?
b. What are the 4 most important steps in the management of this child?
c. Write fluid therapy for first 24 hours for this child.

Q15. A 2½-year-old child is evaluated by a neurologist because of difficulty in walking. Neurological examination documents ataxia and mental retardation. The neurologist notes the presence of multiple telangiectasias involving the conjunctiva, ears and antecubital fossae. The child also has a history of multiple respiratory tract infections.

a. What is the likely diagnosis?
b. What is the mode of inheritance for this disease?
c. Give 3 other clinical features of this disease.
d. Immunoglobulin studies on the child would most likely demonstrate an absence of which immunoglobulin?

Q16. A child weighing 12 kg is admitted with 25% burns.

a. What is the total volume of fluid and what fluid is required for resuscitation?
b. What is the duration for replacement of this fluid?
c. How is it spaced?
d. Is colloid indicated in this child?
e. When is colloid indicated?

Q17. Match the following.

a.	Physostigmine	i.	Mushroom, INH, ethylene glycol
b.	Pyridoxine	ii.	Diazepam
c.	Diphenylhydramine	iii.	Clonidine
d.	Dimercaptosuccinic acid	iv.	Dystonia
e.	Flumazenil	v.	Beta blocker
f.	Naloxone	vi.	Arsenic
g.	EDTA	vii.	Lead
h.	Glycogen	viii.	Anticholinergic agent

Q18. Answer the following questions on drowning.

a. Define:
   i. Drowning
   ii. Near drowning.
b. List 2 electrolyte disturbances and 1 hematological complication of near drowning.
c. What is the commonest radiological finding?

Q19. Answer the following questions.

a. What is pulse oximetry?
b. What is the principle behind it?
c. Mention three limitations of its use.
d. How does it corelate with PO_2?

Q20. A 6-year-old male child is rushed to casualty at night with chief complaint of altered sensorium and cold peripheries since evening (for last 5 hours). According to the parents, he was playing in the garden and suddenly complained of severe pain at the left dorsum of foot. His condition deteriorated over the next 4 hours. Clinically, child had to be intubated and was found to have tachycardia with frothy secretions in the endotracheal tube and shock. Liver was palpable 3.5 cm below the RCM in midclavicular line and B/L crepts were present in the lungs.

a. What is the most probable diagnosis?
b. What management will you give for pain relief?
c. What is the life-saving measure you will take in this patient (other than airway, breathing and circulation)?
d. What is contraindicated as a treatment modality in this patient?
e. What would be the pressor agent of choice to start with?

Q21. You are sitting in a PHC and a child presents to you with alleged history of snake bite. Local examination seems consistent with snake bite. As per the national protocol for snake bite in children.

a. What is "Do it RIGHT"?
b. What is the standard test for coagulopathy?
c. What is the indication for ASV administration?
d. What will be the initial dose of ASV in a child with severe systemic envenomation?

Q22. Study the photo shown below and answer the given questions.

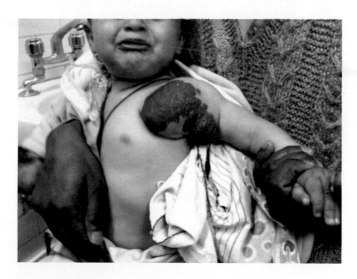

a. What is the best description of this lesion?
b. How do you classify these lesions?

c. Name the immunohistochemical marker that separates hemangiomas from other vascular tumors of infancy.
d. Give two complications of this condition.

Q23. Answer the following questions.
a. Define and elaborate the nerve involved in:
   i. External ophthalmoplegia.
   ii. Internal ophthalmoplegia.
b. Define internuclear ophthalmoplegia and name the tract involved.

Q24. A 2-year-old boy swallowed a hearing aid battery 4 hours back. Chest X-ray done after 4 hours showed battery located in the upper third of the esophagus. Child is playful and stable hemodynamically with no clinical symptomatology. What will be next step in your management and why?

Q25. Answer the following questions.
a. What is dermatoglyphics?
b. What are ulnar loops and what is its significance?
c. What is a triradius and where is it formed?
d. What is the normal 'atd' angle? What happens to the angle in Down's syndrome?
e. What is Sydney line and Kennedy crease?

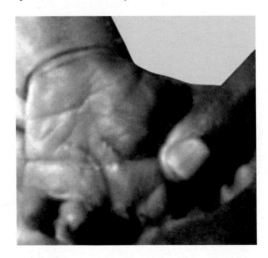

Q26. Answer the following questions on Horner syndrome.
a. What are its components? (Name four).
b. What is the cause for this diagnosis?
c. How do you confirm your diagnosis?

Q27. Study the smear shown below and answer the following questions.

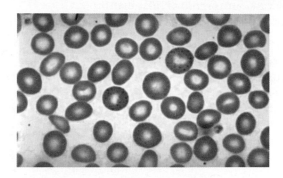

a. Identify the abnormality shown in the smear.
b. Give 2 differential diagnosis for this condition.
c. Describe Porter Index.

Q28. A 4-year-old male child is brought with a history of developmental delay, lethargy and constipation. He is found to have mild mental retardation and sensory neuropathy. He is from low socioeconomic group and his father is a laborer.

a. What is your most probable diagnosis?
b. What test in urine will confirm the diagnosis?
c. What treatment options are available for this condition?
d. What is the indication for treatment for this?

Q29. A 13-year-old, obese boy has been complaining of persistent knee pain and has developed a limp for several weeks. Physical examination of the knee is normal, but shows limited hip motion on the left. As the hip is flexed, the leg goes into external rotation and cannot be rotated internally.

a. What is the most likely diagnosis?
b. What characteristic sign is seen on X-ray of pelvis?
c. Mention two most serious complications of this condition.

Q30. Study the photo below and answer the questions.

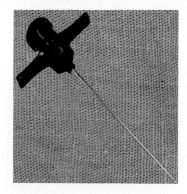

a. What is this instrument?
b. Name the procedure for which this instrument is used.
c. What is the minimum platelet count to be kept prior to this procedure?

Q31. You are working in the emergency department and a 4-year-old child is brought in with severe abdominal pain and back pain with vomiting. On examination, he has generalized tenderness over the abdomen with guarding. You learn he was recently diagnosed with acute lymphoblastic leukemia. His lab investigations showed serum Ca^{+2} 10.8 mEq/L, glucose 420 mg/dL and 3+ ketones in the urine. This child has received vincristine, L-asparaginase, and high dose prednisone.

a. What is your differential diagnosis for the acute problem?
b. How would you manage this?

Q 32. This 7-year-old boy, born of a consanguineous marriage was brought with history of progressive darkening of the skin, nails and teeth, noted by the parents since infancy. The child was unable to tolerate exposure to sunlight due to pain on exposure. Clinically, he was pale, with brownish discoloration of the skin, sclera, teeth, and nails. Liver and spleen were palpable 6 cm and 5 cm below the costal margin. Investigations revealed a hemoglobin of 6 g/dL, with a serum bilirubin (indirect) of 1.8 mg/dL.

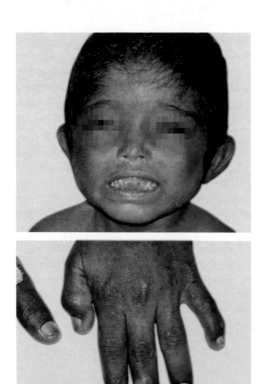

a. What is the most probable diagnosis?
b. What is the screening investigation that you will perform?
c. Name three other causes of generalized skin darkening other than excessive sun exposure.
d. Name three drugs that can cause an acute life-threatening crisis in this child.

Q33. A 10-year-old presents to pediatric OPD with these painful, hot lesions on both shins.

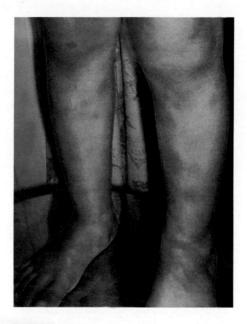

a. What is the diagnosis?
b. List 5 conditions which may be associated with this diagnosis.

ANSWERS

A 1:

a. Should not exceed 40 dB
b. Should not exceed 20 dB
c. 200 sq feet
d. Minimum 3m
e. 8–12 beds
f. 1:1, 1:2.

A 2:

a. Ellis Class 1: Fracture involving enamel
   Ellis Class 2: Fracture involving enamel and dentin
   Ellis Class 3: Fracture involving enamel, dentin and pulp
b. 4 year old: no attempt of reimplantation
   14 year old: Reimplantation as soon as possible
c. Hank's Solution
   Milk
   Underneath patients tongue- provided patient is able to keep from aspiration.

A 3:

	Site of sample collection	Earliest Gestation age to perform the test
CVS or CVB	Small piece of placenta	11 weeks
Amniocentesis	Amniotic fluid	15 weeks
Cordocentesis	Fetal blood	18 weeks

A 4:

a. No
b. No
c. Yes
d. Yes
e. No

A 5:

a. The Guedel airway
b. Maintain a patent airway
c. Size is equal to distance between the lips (or incisors) and the tip to the angle of the jaw
d. Inserted into the patient's mouth upside down: Once contact is made with the back of the throat, the airway is rotated 180 degrees
e. Can be inserted right side up
   Gag reflex and induced vomiting
   Obstruction of airway if size too big
   Damage to teeth.

A 6:

a. Chediak: Higashi syndrome
b. Autosomal recessive. Mutated gene- CHS1 gene
c. Peripheral neuropathy and ataxia
d. Non specific: High-dose ascorbic acid.

A 7:

a. 4
b. 3
c. 5
d. 5

A 8:

a. Grade 4: Clubbing
b. Grade 1: Fluctuation and softening of the nail bed
   Grade 2: Obliteration of normal angle between nail and nail bed
   Grade 3: Accentuated convexity of the nail; drumstick appearance
   Grade 4: Broadened terminal pulp of the digit; pulmonary osteoarthropathy.

A 9:

a. Amrinone.
b. Rate of infusion of the drug (amrinone) and duration of therapy.
c. Phosphodiesterase inhibitor.
d. Increases cellular levels of cAMP.

A 10:

a. Give 10 mL/kg fluid.
b. Pyrethroids.
c. Exchange transfusion.
d. Hydrocarbon and organophosphates.

A 11:

a. Observe the child for at least 6 hours.
b. Preferably after 6 hours.
c. Prophylactic antibiotics should not be given as bacterial pneumonia occurs in very small percentage of cases.
d. Aspiration pneumonitis.

A 12:

a. Urinary retention (in fact urinary incontinence occurs).
b. Atropine and pralidoxime.
c. Accumulation of acetyl choline at peripheral nicotinic and muscarinic synapses in CNS.
d. D – diarrhea/defecation
   U – urination
   M – miosis

B   –   bronchorrhea
B   –   bradycardia
E   –   emesis
L   –   lacrymation
S   –   salivation.

A 13:

a. Cholinergic (organophosphorus) toxicity.
b. Organophosphates and carbamates.
c. Air way, breathing, circulation.
   Gastric lavage/activated charcoal.
   Atropine.
   PAM.
d. Peripheral neuropathy.

A 14:

a. Airway obstruction and inhalational injury (Singed nasal hairs, carbonaceous material in throat, hoarseness of voice, persistent cough, stridor).
b. • Air way, breathing, circulation
   • I/V access and fluids
   • Pain management
   • Management of hypothermia.
c. Parkland formula: Ringer lactate (4 mL/kg/% burn) + Maintenance fluids.

A 15:

a. Ataxia telangiectasia.
b. Autosomal recessive.
c. Choreoathetoid movements, slurred speech, ophthalmoplegia, sinopulmonary infections, cutaneous anergy, endocrine disorders, leukemias, gastric cancers, brain tumors.
d. IgA and IgE.

A 16:

a. 3300 mL of ringer lactate.
b. 24 hours.
c. 50% in the first 8 hours.
   50% in the next 16 hours.
d. No
e. Burns more than 85% BSA; started after 8–24 hours of injury.

A 17:

a. Physostigmine   : Lead
b. Pyridoxine   : Mushroom, INH, ethylene glycol
c. Diphenylhydramine   : Dystonia
d. Dimercaptosuccinic acid : Arsenic
e. Flumazenil   : Diazepam

f. Naloxone   : Clonidine
g. EDTA   : Anticholinergic agent
h. Glycogen   : Beta blocker

A 18:

a. i. Process of experiencing respiratory impairment from submersion or immersion in liquid. The outcome may be death, survival with morbidity or survival without morbidity.
    ii. Any survival from an immersion event.
b. Electrolyte:
    • Hypernatremia
    • Hyperkalemia
    • Hypercalcemia
    • Hypermagnesemia.
Hematological:
    • Hemolysis
Pulmonary edema

A 19:

a. Pulse oximetry is a non-invasive method of measuring the oxygen saturation of hemoglobin in arterial blood.
b. Red and infrared light of different wavelengths when transmitted through the capillary have differential absorption by oxyhemoglobin and reduced hemoglobin. This ratio is then detected by a transducer and displayed as oxygen saturation.
c. False values occur in:
    i.   Poor perfusion
    ii. Ambient light
    iii. Presence of carboxy hemoglobin/methemoglobin
    iv. Movement
d. As per the oxyhemoglobin dissociation curve.

A 20:

a. Scorpion sting with autonomic dysfunction.
b. Xylocaine for local infiltration (if wound identified) and ice application.
c. Prazocin (30 mic/kg at 0, 6, 12 and 24 hours irrespective of blood pressure).
d. Digoxin for CHF.
e. Dobutamine infusion.

A 21:

a. R   =   Reassurance.
    I   =   Immobilize the limb (as in fracture, do not put tourniquet).
    G H =   Get hospitalized.
    T   =   Tell the doctor regarding any symptoms (e.g. ptosis).
b. The 20 minute whole blood clotting test (20 WBCT) is adopted as the standard test for coagulopathy in snake bites.

c. The only indication is systemic envenomation (altered 20 WBCT, or spontaneous bleeding or any neurological impairment).

d. 8–10 vials in any case of systemic envenomation.

A 22:

a. Hemangioma.

b. Superficial, deep and mixed.

c. GLUT-1.

d. Ulceration, secondary infection, hemorrhage.

A 23:

a.   i. External = Extraocular muscle palsy due to 3rd, 4th or 6th nerve palsy.

  ii. Internal = 3rd nerve palsy (sphincter pupillae and ciliaris muscle palsy); Pupil fixed and dilated (no light, consensual or accommodation reflex).

b. Internuclear = Lesion between midbrain and pons, so there will be lesion in the medial longitudinal bundle leading to palsy of conjugate movement.

A 24: Immediate esophagoscopy to retrieve the battery. Hearing aid batteries are highly corrosive and must be removed as early as possible.

A 25:

a. Dermatoglyphics are the configuration formed by fine ridges, on the palmar surface of the hands and fingers.

b. Ulnar loop is formed by ridges entering and leaving the skin surface over the finger tip on the ulnar side.

c. Tri radius is formed at the junction of three sets of converging epidermal ridges, normally tri radii are formed on the palm beneath each finger and in axial plane of palm.

d. Atd angle: Normally = 40°; In Down's syndrome ~ 75° or more.

e. Sydney line: Two transverse crease in palm, proximal extends from radial to ulnar border.

  Kennedy crease: Deep sole crease between the first and second toe.

A 26:

a. • Partial ptosis.
  • Miosis.
  • Anhidrosis.
  • Enophthalmos.
  • If paralysis of ocular sympathetic fibres occurs before 2 years of age, heterochromia iridis with hypopigmentation of iris may occur on the affected side.

b. Sympathetic denervation of eyes (lesions of superior cervical ganglion or sympathetic trunk).

c. **Cocaine test**—Normal pupil dilates within 20–45 minutes after instillation of 1–2 drops of 4% cocaine whereas the miotic pupil of an oculosympathetic paresis dialates poorly, if at all with cocaine.

A 27:

a. Basophilic stippling.

b. – Thalassemia
   – Lead poisoning.
c. The desferal therapeutic index or porter index is defined as mean daily dose of desferrioxamine in mg/kg, divided by serum ferritin.
   – This is calculated every 6 months in patients receiving desferroxamine
   – Porter index should not exceed 0.025 in order to minimize sensorineural hearing loss

A 28:

a. Lead poisoning.
b. Coproporphyrin in urine (CPU) > 150 mic/L.
   Aminolevulinic acid in urine (ALAU) > 5 mg/L.
c. $CaNa_2$ EDTA (calcium versanate) and BAL in symptomatic child.
d. If lead levels > 45 µgm% (Normally < 10 µgm%).

A 29:

a. Slipped capital femoral epiphysis.
b. 'Blanch sign of Steel' on AP view of pelvis (double density created from anteriorly displaced femoral neck overlying the femoral head).
c. Osteonecrosis (avascular necrosis) and chondrolysis.

A 30:

a. Jamshedi bone marrow biopsy needle.
b. Bone marrow biopsy.
c. No cut off for platelets needed prior to bone marrow study.

A 31:

a. Acute pancreatitis with diabetic ketoacidosis.
b. Pain relief, send lipase/amylase and USG abdomen to confirm, start treatment for DKA–IV fluids, insulin, etc. watch for shock. Stop offending drugs asparginase and prednisolone.

A 32:

a. Porphyria (congenital erythropoietic porphyria).
b. Urine for porphobilinogen.
c. Generalized darkening of skin: Addison's disease, hemochromatosis, pregnancy (facial), phototherapy in a case of obstructive jaundice, oral contraceptive.
d. Phenobarbitone, sulphomides, phenytoin, carbamazepine, metoclopramide, rifampicin.

A 33:

a. Erythema nodosum
b. Infections:

Bacterial	– *Streptococcus,* TB, *Salmonella*
Viral	– EBV, HBV
Fungal	– Histoplasma
Inflammatory bowel disease	– Crohns, ulcerative colitis
Autoimmune	– SLE, Behçet, sarcoidosis
Drugs	– Sulphonamides.

Chapter 15

Cardiovascular System

QUESTIONS

Q1. Calculate the heart rate

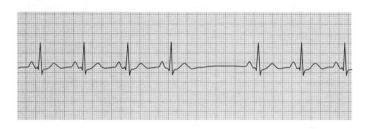

Q2. Is this ECG normal or not? If not why?

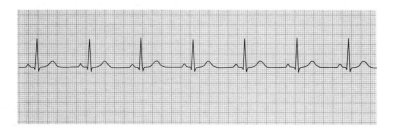

Q3. What is your management?

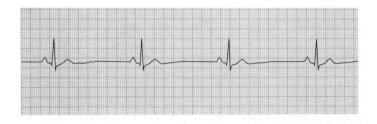

Q4. What is your management?

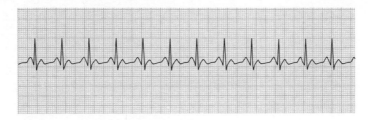

Q5. What is your management?

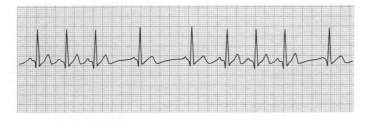

Q6. What is your diagnosis?

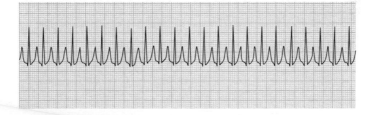

Q7. What is your diagnosis?

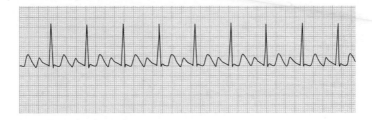

Q8. What is your diagnosis?

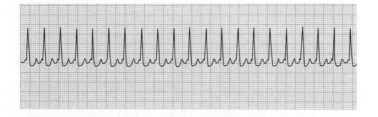

Q9. What is your diagnosis?

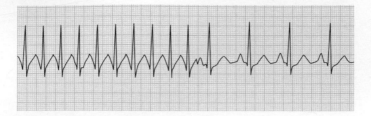

Q10. What is your diagnosis?

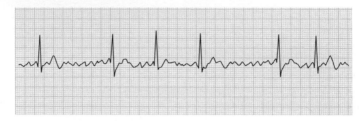

Q11. What is your diagnosis?

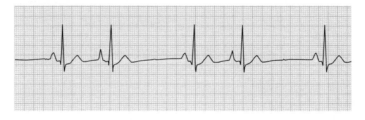

Q12. What is your diagnosis?

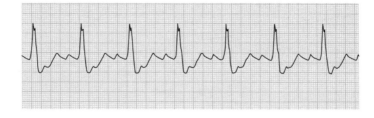

Q13. What is your diagnosis?

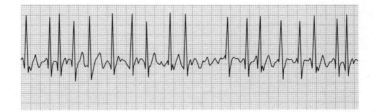

Q14. What is your diagnosis?

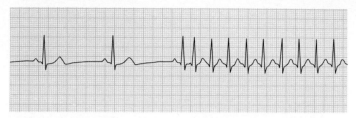

Q15. What is your diagnosis?

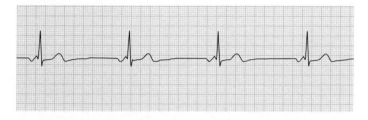

Q16. What is your diagnosis?

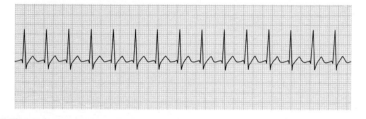

Q17. What does this indicate?

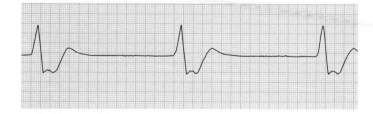

Q18. What is the most common cause?

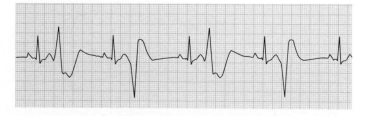

Q19. What is the diagnosis?

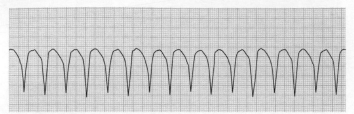

Q20. What is the diagnosis?

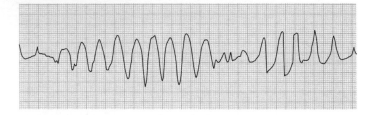

Q21. What is the treatment?

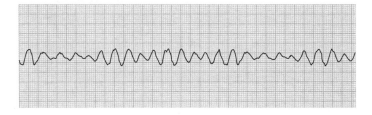

Q22. Could the child be alive?

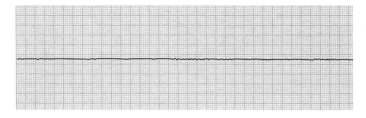

Q23. Is this ECG normal? Why?

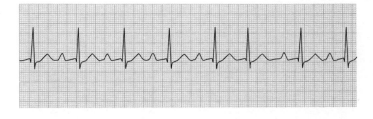

Q24. What is the diagnosis?

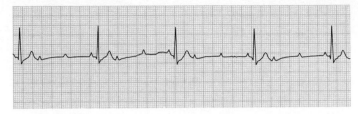

Q25. What is the diagnosis?

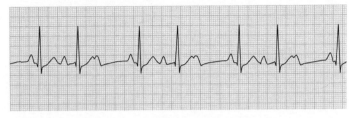

Q26. What is the diagnosis?

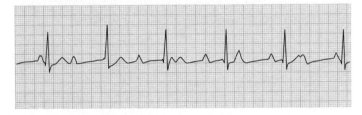

Q27. What is the diagnosis?

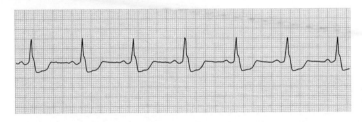

Q28. What is abnormal with this ECG?

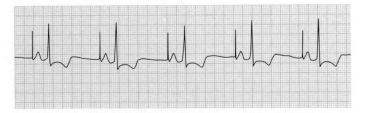

Q29. What is the diagnosis?

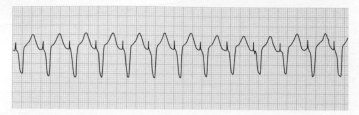

Q30. Healthy child has this ECG. What is the possible cause?

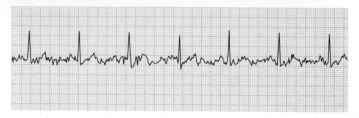

Q31. A 8-year-old male is brought with history of sudden onset giddiness and fall, from which he recovered in a few seconds. His clinical examination was noted to be normal and his ECG is attached below.

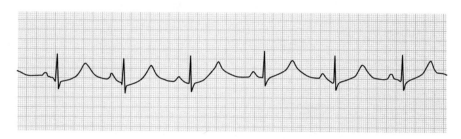

a. Identify this ECG.
b. What is the complication associated with this condition?
c. What is the drug of choice for this diagnosis?
d. Enlist 2 non-pharmacological treatments for the same.

Q32. Match the following.

Inherited condition	Heart abnormality
a. Down syndrome	i. Supravalvular aortic stenosis
b. Turner syndrome	ii. Hypertrophic cardiomyopathy
c. DiGeorge syndrome	iii. Cardiac rhabdomyoma
d. Marfan syndrome	iv. AVSD
e. William syndrome	v. Coarctation of aorta

Contd..

Contd..

f. Tuberous sclerosis	vi. Dissecting aortic aneurysm
g. Pompe disease	vii. Aortic arch abnormality

Q33. ECG diagnosis.

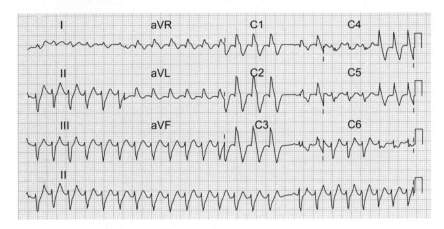

a. What is the ECG diagnosis?
   Patients' pulse cannot be palpated
b. What is the immediate management after initial stabilization?
c. List four etiological causes of pulseless electrical activity (electrical-mechanical-dissociation).

Q34. Please write the ECG event (waves and intervals) related to following cardiac event.

For example, p wave—atrial depolarization:
a. Ventricular depolarization.
b. Ventricular repolarization.
c. Start of atrial depolarization to start of ventricular depolarization.
d. Pause in ventricular activity before repolarization.
e. Total time taken by ventricular depolarization and repolarization.

Q35. You examine a 4-month-old infant in your OPD. Baby was born at term to a primigravida mother with no antenatal concerns. The pediatrician hears a continuous murmur at the upper left sternal border. The peripheral pulses in all extremities are full and show widened pulse pressure.

a. Which is the most likely diagnosis?
b. Name a congenital infection which may be associated with this problem.
c. What is the treatment for this infant?
d. List two other causes of continuous murmur.

Q36. Match the following.

Heart sounds	Associated disease / Cardiac abnormality
a. Loud S_1	i. Pulmonary valve stenosis
b. Soft S_1	ii. Aortic regurgitation
c. Loud P_2	iii. Aortic stenosis
d. Soft P_2	iv. Thyrotoxicosis
e. Reverse splitting of S_2	v. Pulmonary hypertension
f. S_3	vi. Mitral stenosis

Q37. A 6-week-old male infant is seen in pediatric emergency with an episode of cyanosis. Mother complains of similar episodes when the child wakes up in the morning or while crying. On examination the child is still cyanosed and has an ejection murmur heard over upper left sternal border and a single second heart sound.

a. What is the most likely diagnosis?
b. List three common syndrome/associations which can be associated with this condition.
c. What is the characteristic ECG finding of this condition?
   The child has been stabilized in the emergency room.
d. What is the surgical treatment for this abnormality?

Q38. Study the ECG and answer the questions.

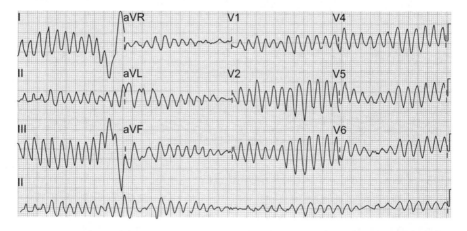

a. What is the diagnosis?
b. What is the treatment?

Q39. A 10-year-old female child presents to pediatric OPD with decreased exercise tolerance. She is noted to have a grade three ejection systolic murmur best heard at the left upper sternal border and a grade three mid diastolic murmur at the lower left sternal border. The second heart sound is widely split and fixed. A right ventricular impulse is palpated.

a. What is the most likely diagnosis?
b. List 3 ECG finding of the commonest type of this abnormality.
c. What is the definitive treatment of this abnormality?
d. Is prophylaxis for infective endocarditis indicated?
e. Name the syndrome associated with this heart condition caused by abnormality of the chromosomal 12.

Q40. An 8-year-old child is seen by a pediatrician for a murmur. The pediatrician hears a loud systolic ejection murmur with a prominent systolic ejection click. The murmur decreases with the Valsalva maneuver. Both murmurs are heard best at the upper right sternal border.

a. What is the most likely diagnosis?
b. What is the ECG finding of this condition?
c. What is the treatment for this abnormality?
d. Name two conditions in which the murmur increases with the Valsalva maneuver.

Q41. A sick 4-year-old is admitted in PICU for bilateral pneumonia. He is nil by mouth and is on ringer lactate. His electrolytes reveal Na 132 and K 8.5. An ECG is ordered.

a. Enlist 4 ECG findings you would expect in this child.
b. Enlist 3 steps in managing this patient.
c. Outline the importance of interpretation of trans tubular potassium gradient (TTKG).

Q42. An 8-month-old female infant presents to pediatric OPD with complaint of poor weight gain. She had 3 episodes of LRTI in past 3 months. On examination, there is a pansystolic murmur heard over the left lower sternal border accompanied by a thrill.

a. What is the most likely cardiac diagnosis?
b. Enlist two differential diagnosis of pansystolic murmur.
c. What is the most common type based on location of the defect?
d. If this baby develops an associated early diastolic murmur with bounding pulses, what is the most likely location of the lesion?
e. Is a loud harsh, holosystolic murmur with thrill along the left lower sternal border suggestive of a large lesion in the diagnosis given above?
f. Lack of cardiac enlargement in a left to right shunt signifies the shunt is:
   i. <2:1
   ii. <1.75:1
   iii. <1.5:1
   iv. <1.2:1

g. A mid diastolic murmur at the mitral area suggests a shunt of:
   i. >1.2:1
   ii. >1.5:1
   iii. >1.75:1
   iv. >2:1

Q43. Match the following:

Cardiac abnormality	JVP abnormality
a. Pulmonary stenosis	• Cannon a wave
b. Complete heart block	• Giant a wave
c. Tricuspid regurgitation	• Steep y descent
d. Constrictive pericarditis	• Large v wave

Q44. Given below is the chest X-ray of a neonate.

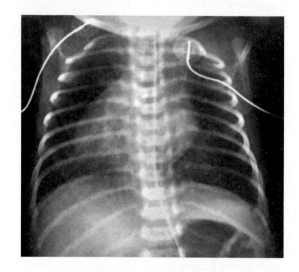

a. What is the most likely radiological diagnosis?
b. List two ECG findings associated with this diagnosis.
c. What should be the placement of pads while defibrillating this patient?

Q45. True false

Physiological (innocent) murmurs.
a. Are heard in a small minority of children.
b. Characteristically change in intensity with the position of the patient.
c. Are more common in infants, who are small for their gestational age.
d. May be associated with a thrill.

Q46. Cardiac device.

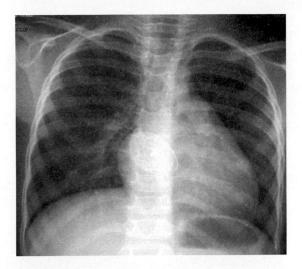

a. Identify the procedure, where the device shown in this X-ray is used.
b. List two indications of this procedure.
c. What is the long-term non-cardiac complication, which may occur, if the device is not placed in asymptomatic children?

Q47. Cardiac device.

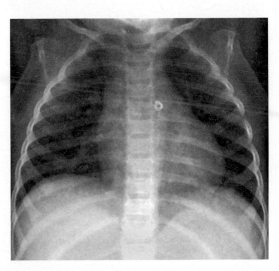

a. Identify the procedure, where the device shown in this X-ray is used.
b. List five complications, which may occur, if the device is not placed in children with the above diagnosis.

ANSWERS

A 1. 60/minute.

A 2. It's a normal ECG (depends on which lead it represents).

A 3. Sinus bradycardia—medical management. Rule out hypothyroidism.

A 4. Sinus tachycardia—rule out hyperthyroidism, febrile illness, anemia and myocarditis.

A 5. Medical management—beta blockers if symptomatic with palpitations.

A 6. Narrow QRS tachycardia—supraventricular tachycardia.

A 7. Sinus tachycardia.

A 8. Supraventricular tachycardia—? atrial flutter.

A 9. Termination of narrow QRS supraventricular tachycardia.

A 10. Atrial fibrillation.

A 11. Atrial ectopic with pause.

A 12. Broad QRS rhythm—needs complete 12 lead ECG

A 13. Atrial fibrillation.

A 14. Onset of atrial fibrillation.

A 15. Low atrial rhythm (negative P waves).

A 16. Supraventricular tachycardia.

A 17. Sinus arrest with broad QRS complex.

A 18. Polymorphic ventricular bigeminy.

A 19. Broad QRS tachycardia—D/D ventricular tachycardia or Supraventricular tachycardia with aberrancy.

A 20. Torsades de pointes.

A 21. Immediate cardioversion and CPR.

A 22. Yes, Hypothermia.

A 23. First degree heart block – prolonged PR.

A 24. 3:1 AV block with narrow QRS escape.

A 25. AV Wenckebach phenomenon.

A 26. Type 2, IInd degree AV block.

A 27. Horizontal ST depression

A 28. Atrial pacing.

A 29. Ventricular paced rhythm.

A 30. Muscle artefact: DDs—improper contact, hypothermia, shivering.

A 31:

a. Prolonged QT syndrome.
b. Torsades de pointes (polymorphic ventricular tachycardia).
c. β blocker-propranolol:
d. • Pace maker
   • Implanted defibrillator.

A 32:

Inherited Condition	Heart abnormality
a. Down syndrome	• AVSD
b. Turner syndrome	• Coarctation of aorta
c. Di George syndrome	• Aortic arch abnormality
d. Marfan syndrome	• Dissecting aortic aneurysm
e. William syndrome	• Supravalvular aortic stenosis
f. Tuberous sclerosis	• Cardiac rhabdomyoma
g. Pompe disease	• Hypertrophic cardiomyopathy

A 33:

a. Ventricular tachycardia, immediate treatment.
b. Defibrillation.
c. Hyperkalemia, hypothermia, hypovolemia, tension pneumothorax, hypoxia, pericardial tamponade, toxins, pulmonary thromboembolism.

A 34:

a. QRS complex
b. T wave
c. PR interval
d. ST segment
e. QT interval.

A 35:
a. Patent ductus arteriosus
b. Congenital rubella infection
c. Surgical/coil ligation
d. Aortico pulmonary window defect:
   Cervical venous hum
   Ruptured sinus of valsalva aneurysm
   Coronary AV fistula
   Truncus arteriosus with increased pulmonary flow.

A 36:

Heart sounds	Associated disease Cardiac abnormality
a. Loud S_1	• Thyrotoxicosis
b. Soft S_1	• Mitral stenosis
c. Loud P_2	• Pulmonary hypertension
d. Soft P_2	• Pulmonary valve stenosis
e. Reverse splitting of S_2	• Aortic stenosis
f. S_3	• Aortic regurgitation

A 37:
a. Tetralogy of Fallot (cyanotic spells).
b. Down syndrome:
   DiGeorge syndrome
   CHARGE
   VACTERL
c. RAD
   RVH
d. Palliative BT shunt within few months of life
   Corrective surgery at 4 to 12 months age.

A 38:
a. Torsades de pointes
b. β-blocker-propranolol
   Pace maker
   Implanted defibrillator

A 39:
a. ASD
b. RAD
   RSR pattern in right precordial leads or RBBB
   RVH.
c. Device closure/surgical closure.
d. Not indicated.
e. Holt Oram syndrome.

A 40:

a. Aortic valve stenosis.
b. LVH with strain pattern (inverted T wave in left precordial leads).
c. Balloon valutoplasty or aortic valve replacement.
d. Hypertrophic obstructive cardiomyopathy and mitral valve prolapse.

A 41:

a. Peaking of the T waves.
 Increased P-R interval.
 Flattening of the P wave.
 Widening of the QRS complex.
b. Stop all sources of additional potassium
 Calcium
 Combination of insulin and glucose
 Bicarbonate (most efficacious in a patient with a metabolic acidosis)
 Sodium polystyrene sulfonate (K exchange resin)
 Dialysis.
c. $\dfrac{(K)\ \text{Urine}\ \times\ \text{Plasma osmolality}}{(K)\ \text{Plasma}\ \times\ \text{Urine osmolality}}$

 If TTKG in Hyperkalemic patient is < 8 then likely cause is renal.

A 42:

a. VSD
b. MR TR
c. Membranous
d. Supracristal region
e. No
f. <1.75:1
g. >2:1

A 43:

Cardiac abnormality	JVP abnormality
a. Pulmonary stenosis	• Giant a wave
b. Complete heart block	• Cannon a wave
c. Tricuspid regurgitation	• Large v wave
d. Constrictive pericarditis	• Steep y descent

A 44:

a. Dextrocardia with situs solitus.
b. Inverted P wave.
 Inverted T wave.
 QRS Complex is negative in lead I
 Lead II and III are reversed from normal appearance
 Lead II resembles a normal lead III
 Lead III resembles a normal lead II.

c. Instead of upper right and lower left, pads should be placed upper left and lower right.

A 45:

a. False
b. True
c. False
d. False.

A 46:

a. ASD device closure
b. All symptomatic patients:
   Asymptomatic patients with a Qp : Qs ratio of at least 2 : 1
c. Paradoxical (right to left) systemic embolization.

A 47:

a. PDA coil closure
b. Cardiac failure:
   Infective endarteritis
   Aneurysmal dilatation of the pulmonary artery or the ductus
   Calcification of the ductus
   Non-infective thrombosis of the ductus with embolization
   Paradoxical emboli
   Pulmonary hypertension.

Chapter

16

Growth, Development and Nutrition

QUESTIONS

Q1. Select the answers.

a. Measure development of a 1-year-old
b. Measure intelligence of a 10-year-old
c. Detection of hemiparesis in a 3-month-old
d. Detection of blindness or deafness in 2-month-old
    i. Clinical neurological examination
    ii. Electroencephalogram
    iii. Gesell schedules
    iv. Thematic apperception test (TAT)
    v. Wechsler intelligence scale (WISC) test.

Q2. Select the answers.

a. Suicidal behavior
b. Gender identity
c. Oedipal years
d. Latency
    i. 0–2 years
    ii. 3–6 years
    iii. 6–12 years
    iv. 12–14 years
    v. 14–16 years.

Q3. For each description of development accomplishments, select the earliest most appropriate age.

a. Walk if led and is able to talk a few steps unsupported, demonstrates a good pincer grip, drinks from a cup.
b. Copies a circle, hold on one foot, recognizes colors.
c. Smiles responsively, follows a moving object or face with turning of the head.
d. Kicks a ball, builds a tower of six 1-in cubes, combines two different words.

e. Sits without support, pulls to a stand, babbles loudly and happily, grabs a block with the entire hand.
f. Startles at sudden noise.
g. Draws a triangles, uses past and future tense in language.
  i. 2 Months
  ii. 4 Months
  iii. 6 Months
  vi. 9 Months
  v. 12 Months
  vi. 18 Months
  vii. 2 Years
  viii. 3–4 Years
  ix. 5 Years.

Q4. Nutrition reserve in adult and children—survival without food.

How long can a given subject survive without food?
a. Adults
b. 1 year old
c. Term infant
d. Preterm infant 2 kg
e. Preterm infant 1 kg
  Choose from options below.
  i. 1 year
  ii. 6 months
  iii. 3 months
  iv. 90 days
  v. 45 days
  vi. 30 days
  vii. 12 days
  viii. 4 days
  ix. 1 day
  x. 12 hours
  xi. 1 hour.

Q5. The following food substances, which contain vitamin A, need to be arranged based on vitamin A content from low to high.

a. Papaya
b. Guava
c. Drumstick leaves
d. Egg
e. Human milk
f. Carrot.

Q6. Write the calorie value of

a. Rice—1 cup
b. Puri—1
c. Upma—1 cup

d. Idli—1
e. Dosa—1
f. Kichidi—1 cup
g. Boiled egg—1
h. Vada—1
i. Pizza—1 slice
j. Oil—1 tbsp
k. Ice cream—½ cup
l. Peanuts—50 nos
m. Banana—1
n. Cashew nuts—10
o. Milk chocolate—25 g.

Q7. A 6-year-old girl comes in OPD with complain of difficulty in vision. The child has a history of recurrent episodes of loose stools and pneumonias. Her weight is 8 kg and height is 82 cm. Her eye examination findings are shown below.

Study the photograph and answer the questions:

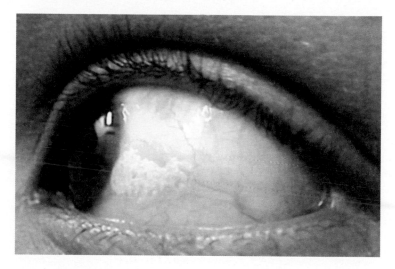

a. What is the positive finding seen in the photograph?
b. What is the most likely diagnosis?
c. Enumerate the WHO staging.
d. What is the staging of the disease in this child?
e. How can you treat this problem at early stages?

Q8. Answer the following questions.
a. What are WHO-MGRS charts?
b. List 2 exclusion criteria used in these charts.
c. List 2 advantages of these charts over the CDC/NCHS charts.

Q9. Waterlow classification of malnutrition.

An 8-year-old boy is noted to have weight of 67% of expected and height of 83% of expected.

a.   What is the degree of malnutrition according to Waterlow Classification?

b.   Give details of Waterlow classification of malnutrition.

Q10. The IQ of a 7-year-old child is 40.

a.   What is his degree of severity of mental retardation?

b.   How do you classify MR on basis of degree of severity?

Q11. Gomez classification of malnutrition.

A 6-year-old boy is noted to have a weight of 61% of expected and height of 90% of expected.

a.   What is the degree of malnutrition according to Gomez classification?

b.   Give details of Gomez classification of malnutrition.

c.   How do you define mild, moderate and severe malnutrition according to Gomez classification?

Q12. At what age does child copy following figures.

a. Square

b.   Circle

c.   Diamond

d.   Vertical stroke   _____

Q13. A 9-month-old girl is seen in paediatric OPD for routine measles immunization. She is noted to have a large head with head circumference plotting above 91st centile. During her previous visit her head circumference has been between 75th to 91st centile. Her weight and height is plotted on 50th centile. She is standing with support with no obvious developmental concerns. There are no parental concerns. Her systemic and neurological

examination is entirely normal.

a. Is there reason to be concerned about this child's head growth?
b. What physical findings not present in this case might suggest serious pathology?
c. What is the next step in the evaluation of this baby?
d. What is the most likely diagnosis?
e. What are some additional differential consideration?

Q14. A 10-year-old boy is seen in pediatric OPD with parental concerns of being under weight. He has a weight of 39.2 kg and a height of 140 cm.

a. What is the formula for calculating BMI?
b. Calculate the BMI of this child.
c. What is your impression about this child's BMI?

Q15. Given below is the BMI centile chart for boys.

Based on the chart below define:

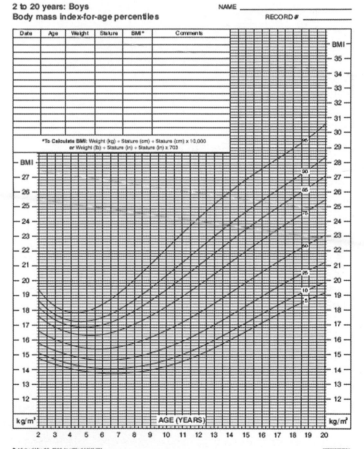

2 to 20 years: Boys
Body mass index-for-age percentiles

a. Underweight
b. Normal weight
c. At risk for overweight
d. Overweight.

Q16. Wellcome classification of malnutrition.

A 5-year-old boy is noted to have a weight of 70% of expected and height of 93% of expected. There is no edema.

a. What is the degree of malnutrition according to Wellcome classification?
b. Give details of Wellcome classification of malnutrition.

Q17. A 14-year-old boy is brought to pediatric OPD with concerns of delayed puberty. On examination, he has preadolescent male genitalia with scanty axillary hairs, and few fine pubic hairs.

a. What is the tanner staging of this child?
   i. Stage 1–2
   ii. Stage 2–3
   iii. Stage 3–4
   iv. Stage 4–5
b. What is the first visible sign of puberty in males?
c. At what tanner stage does a male child achieve peak growth velocity?
   i. Stage 1–2
   ii. Stage 2–3
   iii. Stage 3–4
   iv. Stage 4–5.

Q18. A 11-year-old girl is brought to pediatric OPD with concerns of early signs of puberty. On examination, she has well formed breasts with areola and papilla forming a secondary mound and projecting nipples. She has adult distribution pubic hairs.

a. What is the tanner staging of this child?
b. What is the first visible sign of puberty in females?
c. At what tanner stage does the female attain menarche?
d. Define precocious puberty in girls and boys.

Q19. A 14-month-old male toddler is brought to a pediatrician with parental concerns of delayed eruption of tooth.

a. What is delayed tooth eruption?
b. List 2 common causes.
c. Which is commonly the first tooth to appear?
d. At what age are the following deciduous teeth shed:
   i. First molar.
   ii. Maxillary central incisors.

Q20. Match the following micronutrient with their effects of deficiency.

Micronutrient	Effects of deficiency
a. Selenium	i. Hypercholesterolemia
b. Manganese	ii. Impaired glucose tolerance
c. Fluoride	iii. Night blindness
d. Chromium	iv. Dental caries
e. Molybdenum	v. Cardiomyopathy

Q21. IAP Classification of malnutrition.

A 3-year-old girl is noted have a weight of 55% of expected and height of 91% of expected.

a. What is the degree of malnutrition according to IAP classification?
b. Give details of IAP classification of malnutrition.
c. How do you define severe malnutrition according to IAP classification?

Q22. Fill in the following table regarding developmental reflexes in normal children.

Reflex	Age of appearance	Age of disappearance
Rooting		
Moro		
Landau		
Parachute		

Q23. A 14-year-old girl presents in pediatric OPD clinic with complaint of short stature. Her height is 154 cm. Her mother's height is 156 cm and father's height is 167 cm.

a. What is the formula for calculating the mid parental height for girls?
b. What is the mid parental height for this girl?

Q24. A 2-month-old infant born at 32 weeks gestation is suspected to have vitamin E deficiency.

a. Name two manifestations which will make you think of vitamin E deficiency in this baby.
b. What is the role of vitamin E in humans?
c. How will you diagnose vitamin E deficiency?
d. Give the content of vitamin E in evion drops.

Q25. An 8-month-old boy is reviewed in paediatric OPD for acute gastroenteritis. On detailed history he was noted to have mild developmental delay. No other significant factor was noted in history. On examination, he was noted to have microcephaly. His remaining general and systemic examination was noted to be normal.

a. How do you define microcephaly?
b. List 2 most important investigations for this child.
c. List 4 non-genetic causes of microcephaly.

Q26. A 10-year-old girl presents in pediatric OPD with short stature.

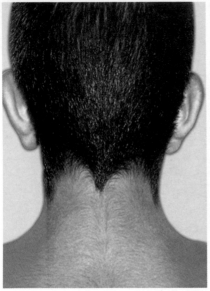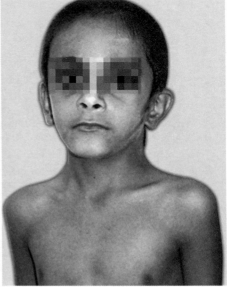

a. List 3 positive findings seen in the photographs.
b. What is the most likely diagnosis?
c. How would you manage her short stature?

ANSWERS

A 1:

a. 3
b. 5
c. 1
d. 1.

A 2:

a. 5
b. 1
c. 2
d. 3.

A 3:

a. 5
b. 8
c. 1
d. 7
e. 4
f. 1
g. 9.

A 4:

a. iii
b. v
c. vii
d. vii
e. viii

A 5:

a.	Guava	0
b.	Human milk	38
c.	Papaya	118
d.	Egg	140
e.	Drumstick leaves	300
f.	Carrot.	1167

A 6:

a.	Rice—1 cup	- 170
b.	Puri—1	- 100
c.	Upma—1 cup	- 270
d.	Idlli—1	- 75
e.	Dosa—1	- 125
f.	Kichidi—1 cup	- 200

g. Boiled egg—1   - 90
h. Vada—1   - 70
i. Pizza—1 slice   - 200
j. Oil—1 tbsp   - 60
k. Ice cream—½ cup   - 200
l. Peanuts—50 nos   - 90
m. Banana—1   - 90
n. Cashew nuts—10   - 95
o. Milk chocolate—25g   - 140

A 7:

a. Bitot's spot.
b. Vitamin A deficiency.
c. WHO staging:

Primary signs
X 1 A   : Conjunctival xerosis
X 1 B   : Bitot's spots
X2   : Corneal xerosis
X3A   : Corneal ulceration (<1/3rd)
X3B   : Keratomalacia.

Secondary signs
XN   : Night blindness
XF   : Xerophthalmia fundus
XS   : Corneal scars.

d. Stage X1B
e. Xerophthalmia is treated by giving 1,500 µg/kg body weight orally for 5 days followed by intramuscular injection of 7,500 µg of vitamin A in oil, until recovery.

A 8:

a. WHO—Multicentric growth reference study charts, developed in 2006.
b. *Exclusion criteria:*
    • Formula fed infants
    • Children of mothers who smoked during or after the pregnancy
    • Morbidities that affect growth (repeated bouts of diarrhea).
c. *Advantages:*
    • The growth charts show how children *should* grow in all countries.
    • MGRS are a *standard* rather than a *reference.*
    • Any deviation from suggested pattern is evidence of abnormal growth.
    • MGRS provide a solid foundation for development of a standard because they are based on healthy children living under condition likely to favor achievement of their full genetic potential.

A 9:

a. Severe wasting and severe stunting.
b. Waterlow classification.

	Weight for height (wasting)	Height for age (stunting)
Normal	> 90	> 95
Mild	80–90	90–95
Moderate	70–80	85–90
Severe	< 70	< 85

A 10:

a. Moderate mental retardation
b. Mild mental retardation   : IQ level 50–55 to > 70
   Moderate mental retardation   : IQ level 35–40 to 50–55
   Severe mental retardation   : IQ level 20–25 to 35–40
   Profound mental retardation   : IQ level below 20–25
   Mental retardation, severity unspecified : When there is a strong presumption of mental retardation but; this is untestable by standard tests.

A 11:

a. Grade 2 malnutrition
b. *Gomez*   *Weight for age (WHO)*
   Normal   >90%
   I degree malnutrition   75–90%
   II degree malnutrition 60–75%
   III degree malnutrition < 60%
c. I degree malnutrition Mild malnutrition
   II degree malnutrition Moderate malnutrition
   III degree malnutrition Severe malnutrition.

A 12:

a. 4 years
b. 3 years
c. 5 years
d. 2 years (imitates at 18 months).

A 13:

a. Yes. The fact that the head size is showing a progressive increase is more concerning than the size alone.
b. 1. Bulging fontanelle
   2. Spread sutures
   3. Lethargy
   4. Neurologic abnormalities: sun-setting of eye, abnormal tone, delayed development
c. Measure head sizes of parents and siblings
d. Familial macrocephaly
e. – Hydrocephalus

– Mucopolysaccharide storage disease
– Syndromic, i.e. Sotos syndrome (cerebral gigantism).

A 14:

a. $\dfrac{\text{Weight in kg}}{(\text{Height in meter})^2}$

b. 20 kg/m²
c. Normal BMI

A 15:

a. Underweight: < 5th percentile.
b. Normal weight: 5th to 84th percentile.
c. At risk for overweight: 85th to 94th percentile.
d. Overweight: > 95th percentile.

A 16:

a. Undernutrition
b. Wellcome classification: evaluates the child for edema and with the Gomez classification system.

Weight for age (Gomez)	With edema	Without edema
60–80%	Kwashiorkor	Undernutrition
< 60%	Marasmic-kwashiorkor	Marasmus

A 17:

a. Stage 1–2.
b. Testicular enlargement.
c. Stage 3–4.

A 18:

a. Stage 5.
b. Appearance of breast buds.
c. Stage 3–4.
d. Precocious puberty is defined as the onset of secondary sexual characteristics before 8 years of age in girls and 9 years in boys.

A 19:

a. Delayed eruption is usually considered when there are no teeth by approximately 13 month of age (mean + 3 standard deviations).
b. Hypothyroidism.
   Hypoparathyroidism
   Familial
   Idiopathic (the most common).
c. Central incisors.
d.   i. 10–12 years
     ii. 7–8 years

A 20:

Micronutrient	Effects of deficiency
a. Selenium	• Cardiomyopathy
b. Manganese	• Hypercholesterolemia
c. Fluoride	• Dental caries
d. Chromium	• Impaired glucose tolerance
e. Molybdenum	• Night blindness

A 21:

a. Grade 3 malnutrition

b.

Grade	Weight for age
Normal	>80%
Grade 1	71–80%
Grade 2	61–70%
Grade 3	51–60%
Grade 4	<50%

c. Grade 3–4

A 22:

Reflex	Age of appearance	Age of disappearance
Rooting	Birth	3 months
Moro	Birth	5-6 months
Landau	10 months	24 months
Parachute	8-9 months	Persists

A 23:

a. $\dfrac{\text{Father Ht} + \text{Mother Ht} - 13}{2}$

b. 155 cm

A 24:

a. Thrombocytosis, edema, hemolysis or anemia.

b. Antioxidant.

c. Vitamin E to serum lipids ratio; a ratio <0.8 mg/g is abnormal.

d. 50 mg/mL.

A 25:

a. Microcephaly is defined as a head circumference that measures more than three standard deviations below the mean for age and sex.

b. CT/MRI.
   TORCH screening.
   Metabolic screening.
   Chromosomal analysis.

c. Congenital infections—CMV, Rubella, Toxoplasmosis.
    Meningitis/encephalitis.
    Hypoxic-ischemic encephalopathy.
    Metabolic.
    Drugs, e.g. fetal alcohol.
    Radiation exposure.

A 26:

a. Low hair line/trident hairline.
    Web neck.
    Widely spaced nipples.
b. Turner syndrome.
c. GH supplementation.

Chapter 17

Neonatology

QUESTIONS

Q1.

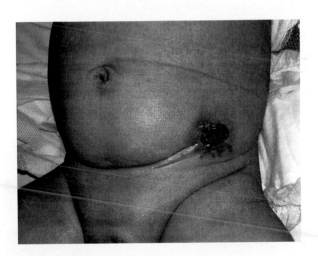

a. What procedure has this patient undergone?
b. Enlist the 2 indication for the procedure.
c. Mention 3 common complications post procedure.
d. What care does the patient need following procedure?

Q2. Select the answers.

a. Can lead to substantial elevations of serum bilirubin
b. Most likely to induce acute hypovolemic shock
c. Drainage is contraindicated
d. Generally resolves by 48 hours of age
   i.   Cephalhematoma
   ii. Caput succedaneum
   iii. Cephalhematoma and caput succedaneum
   iv. Subgaleal hematoma
   v.   Cephalhematoma, caput succedaneum, and subgaleal hematoma

Q3.

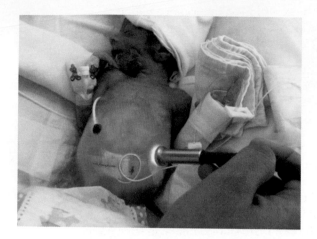

a. What test is being performed in the baby?
b. What is the finding in this baby?
c. What does the finding suggest?
d. What is the treatment?
e. Where else can this test be performed?
f. What can be another use of the equipment?

Q4.

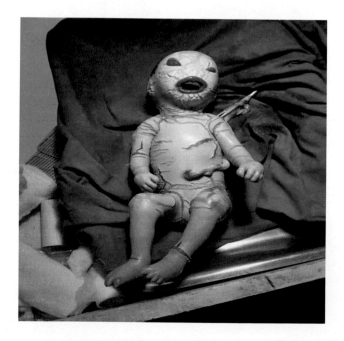

a. What is the diagnosis?
b. What is the incidence?

c. What is the cause?

d. What is the commonest inheritance pattern?

e. What are immediate and long-term complications?

f. What is the treatment?

Q5. 1.2 kg, 7 day old, 28 week newborn is receiving protein at 3 g/kg/day, lipid at 2 g/kg/day and GIR of 6 mg/kg/min. Baby is nil by mouth.

Calculate.

a. NPC/N

b. Fluid rate of below to achieve above goals

   i. 10% protein

   ii. 20% lipid

   iii. 15% dextrose

c. i. Total calorie intake.

   ii. What is the significance of NPC/N and optimal rate?

d. What is the adequate calorie intake in such baby?

Q6. Match the Following:

Teratogens/Maternal Diseases	*Potential Effects/Disorder*
1. Alcohol	A. Arthrogryposis
2. Sodium valproate	B. Long philtrum
3. Diabetics mellitus	C. Neural tube defects
4. Lithium	D. Caudal regression syndrome
5. Myasthenia gravis	E. Ebstein's anomaly

Q7. Study the photograph and answer the questions.

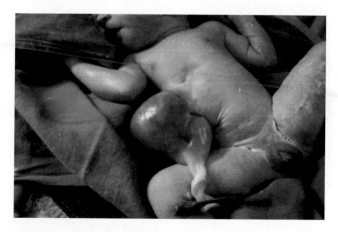

This female neonate was born with a large mass in relation to the umbilical cord:

a. Identify the condition.

b. Give three important aspects that you will take care of in the transport of such a neonate.

c. List 3 anomalies associated with this condition.

d. What is the definitive treatment for this condition?

Q8. A term male baby weighing 3.6 kg presents on day 2 of life with seizures. Mother is gravida 4 with history of 2 neonatal deaths with one live child aged 3 years. He was born at home and mother had a history of greenish vaginal discharge just prior to delivery.

a. Enlist 3 most likely causes of seizures in this baby.
b. Write first 5 steps of management of the current episode of seizure in sequential order.

Q9. You are attending pediatrician of a 31 week preterm whose birth weight was 1400 g. He had an uneventful NICU stay except for 1 day of phototherapy for jaundice.

a. List 3 criteria for discharge?
b. Is this neonate a candidate for:
    i. ROP screening
    ii. Cranial USG
    iii. Hearing screening.

Q10. A HBsAg +ve woman is 20 weeks pregnant.

a. What are the other relevant investigations you would request?
b. The risk of perinatal transmission is maximum if mother is HBe Ag + and
_____.
c. What is the advice to be given to the partner/husband?
d. What is the ideal management of a preterm newborn after birth?

Q11. A term baby is born to a mother via elective cesarian section. The mother is diagnosed to have HIV infection. The baby's test for HIV DNA PCR is positive within 48 hours.

a. What does this positive PCR imply?
b. How would you confirm the diagnosis?
c. What are the drugs used to control? (Name 3 subgroups with 1 example in each group).

Q12. A 5-day-old girl who was delivered at home has presented in emergency for bruising and gastrointestinal bleeding. There is no history of maternal drug or alcohol abuse during pregnancy. There is no family history of similar problems. Laboratory findings are given below.

Haemoglobin	: 15.2 g/dL
Platelet count	: 290,000/mm³
INR	: >2
APTT	: >100 seconds
Serum bilirubin	: 3.5 mg/dL
SGPT	: 41 mg/dL
SGOT	: 28 mg/dL

a. What is the most likely diagnosis of this bleeding neonate?
b. Enlist 2 risk factors in a neonate admitted to NICU which can potentially lead into this problem.

c. How can you prevent the same?

d. How would you treat once the diagnosis is confirmed?

Q13. A term male infant is born via normal vaginal delivery. He is found to have choanal atresia, bilateral colobomas, ear anomalies, and cryptorchidism.

a. What is the most likely diagnosis?

b. What are the 2 problems which are likely to exist in this neonate on further evaluation or later on in the childhood?

c. What is the most appropriate initial test to exclude any associated abnormalities?

d. What is the treatment of choanal atresia in an otherwise stable child?

Q14. A term male newborn delivered at home is seen in the pediatric OPD on day 2 of life.

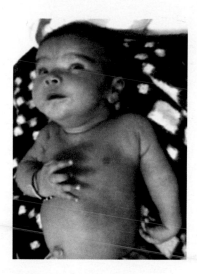

a. What are abnormalities detected in the left arm of this baby?

b. What is the likely diagnosis?

c. What is the etiology?

d. What is the most common associated complication?

Q15. Match the following.

In monozygotic twins what is the relationship between chronicity, amnionicity and timing of division of egg:

Type of chorion and amnion	Timing of division of egg
a. Monochorionic, monoamniotic	(i) 0–3 days
b. Monochorionic, diamniotic	(ii) 3–7 days
c. Dichorionic, diamniotic	(iii) 7–14 days
d. Conjoint twins	(iv) >14 days.

Q16. Given below is CT of an 1800 g term male neonate born to an unbooked primigravida mother.

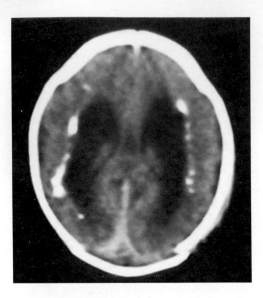

a. List 2 positive findings on the CT.
b. What is the most likely etiological diagnosis?
c. List 2 possible clinical findings in the neonatal period which may accompany the likely diagnosis.

Q17. A 26 week male infant is born via emergency LSCS in view of absent end diastolic flow on umbilical arterial Doppler. The baby is now 3 hours old and has been intubated and ventilated. He has received 1 dose of surfactant. His ventilator settings are:

Mode	CMV
PIP	22 cm H_2O
PEEP	5 cm H_2O
Rate	40/min
FiO_2	30%
Saturation	95%

His arterial blood gas shows

pH	7.18
pCO_2	62 mm Hg
pO_2	78 mm Hg
HCO_3^-	24 mm Hg

a. What are the blood gas findings?
b. What change will you make in the ventilator settings to improve the blood gas?
c. What is the optimal size of ETT for this neonate?

Q18. Given below is the blood gas of a 2 day old 28 week preterm neonate.

Her ventilator settings are:

Mode	SIMV
PIP	21
PEEP	5
Rate	30
FiO_2	21%
Saturation	98%

Her arterial blood gas shows:

pH	7.48
pCO_2	22
pO_2	99
HCO_3^-	29

a. What are the blood gas findings?
b. What changes will you make in the ventilator settings to improve the blood gas?
c. List 2 most important risks/complications which can occur if you leave this baby on current ventilator settings?

Q19. You are an attending resident of a level 3 NICU and are asked to perform a partial exchange transfusion of a preterm female neonate. She is now 12 hours old and weighs 2 kg. Her hematocrit is 80 and desired is 50.

a. What is the formula for calculating volume of partial exchange transfusion?
b. What is the volume required for this neonate?
c. List 3 complications of polycythemia

Q20. You are an attending resident of a level 3 NICU and are asked to review blood gas of a term female infant. She is now 2 hours old and is diagnosed to have meconium aspiration syndrome.

Her ventilator settings are

Mode	CMV
PIP	26
PEEP	3.5
Rate	60
FiO_2	100%
IT	0.5
Saturation	81%

Her arterial blood gas shows

pH	7.41
pCO_2	32
pO_2	51
HCO_3^-	23

a. What is the blood gas finding?
b. What changes will you make in the ventilator settings to improve the blood gas?
c. What is alternate mode of ventilation you can use for this baby?

Q21. A term female infant is born via a difficult instrumental delivery. On examination she is noted to have a wrist drop and paralysis of small muscles of right hand. Her rest of the general and systemic examination is unremarkable.

a. What is the likely diagnosis?
b. What is the etiology?
c. What is the most common associated complication?

Q22. A 26-week-old male infant is born via emergency LSCS. Mother is a primigravida and had no risk factors for sepsis. The baby has been intubated, ventilated and has received 1 dose of surfactant. UAC, UVC and a peripheral cannula have been placed. He is started on IV fluids and IV antibiotics. His Hb is 18, platelet is 250,000. His HR is 170/min, mean BP 23 mm Hg, saturation 92%.

His ventilator settings are:

Mode	CMV
PIP	20
PEEP	5
Rate	40
FiO_2	30%

His arterial blood gas shows:

pH	7.18
pCO_2	39
pO_2	78
HCO_3^-	14

a. What are the blood gas findings?
b. What is the diagnosis?
c. What is the next step in treatment of this neonate?

Q23. Management of cardiogenic shock.

A 12-hour-old 28 weeker is admitted in NICU. She is diagnosed to have respiratory distress syndrome. Her ventilator parameters are currently stable but the staff nurse is concerned about the blood pressure. Her CFT is 3 second, mean BP is 22 mm Hg and CVP is 8 mm Hg. You have already given a fluid bolus of normal saline 30 minute back.

Her arterial blood gas shows

pH	7.20
pCO_2	40
pO_2	68
HCO_3^-	17

a. Enlist the 2 most important drugs you could use in treating hypotension in this patient.
b. What precaution will you take whilst measuring CVP of a baby on ventilator?
c. What is the normal range of CVP?
d. Where should be the tip of UVC to measure CVP?
e. What is the relationship of CVP and volume replacement in managing hypotension?

Q24. A 32-weeks-old male infant is born via normal vaginal delivery. He soon started having moderate respiratory distress with increasing oxygen requirement. A decision is made to start him on nasal CPAP.

a. What is the ideal pressure to start CPAP in this neonate?
b. Enlist three complications associated with nasal CPAP.
c. Enlist two absolute contraindications of nasal CPAP.

Q25. A Sick term male infant is admitted in NICU. He is born to a primigravida mother with no significant antenatal concerns and no risk factors for sepsis. He was born via normal vaginal delivery and did not require any resuscitation. He developed significant respiratory distress soon after birth. He was intubated and ventilated at 2 hours age. He is persistently cyanosed at 4 hours of age. His blood report (including CBC, CRP), chest X-ray have been reported normal. He is currently on high frequency ventilator. His saturation in right lower limb is 76% and right upper limb is 92%. His mean BP is 42 mm Hg and HR is 180/min.

An ECHO has been performed and does not show any structural cardiac abnormality or cyanotic heart disease.

a. What is the most likely diagnosis?
b. What is the drug of choice?
c. What is the best treatment modality if medical management fails?
d. List 4 drugs which can be used in treating this condition.

Q26. A 34 week male infant is born via normal vaginal delivery. He is noted to be jittery and lethargic at 24 hours age. On examination, he is noted to be plethoric.

a. What is the most likely diagnosis?
b. How do you confirm the diagnosis? Give the age related values to confirm the diagnosis at 2 hours and thereafter.
c. What is the treatment if the diagnosis is confirmed in this neonate?

Q27. Given below is the picture of a 2 day old term newborn.

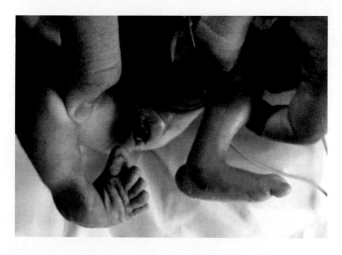

a. What is the diagnosis?
b. List any 2 common risk factors for this problem.
c. List 3 components of this abnormality.
d. What are the treatment options?

Q28. A term male infant was born via elective LSCS to a primigravida mother. He was shifted to NICU in view of hypoglycemia on day 1 of life. His examination revealed a microphallus. On further investigation his free T$_4$ and TSH level were found to be 0.5 µg/dL (normal = 6.5–16.3 µg/dL) and 1.6 mU/L (normal = 1.7-9.1 mU/mL) respectively.

a. What is the most likely diagnosis?
b. List 2 investigations you would perform on this baby.

Q29. A term neonate is diagnosed to have hypothyroidism based on initial routine neonatal screening. He is investigated further and his BERA reveals bilateral sensorineural hearing loss.

a. What is the most likely diagnosis?
b. What is the mode of inheritance?
c. What is the cause of hypothyroidism associated with this diagnosis?
d. What is the finding on thyroid scan and thyroid ultrasound?

Q30. A term neonate was born in poor condition needing prolonged resuscitation. He was born via emergency LSCS for a non reactive NST. At birth he was cyanosed, limp, with HR< 60/min. His condition improved with IPPV. At 1 hour age he is lethargic with diminished spontaneous movements. On examination, he is noted to have mild hypotonia with a weak suck.

a. What is the most likely diagnosis?
b. What is the staging of the disease in this neonate?
c. After what gestation can you use this staging?
d. What is the likely outcome?
e. In neonatal resuscitation—what is the order of recovery in the heart rate, color and tone in most neonates after the initial depression of vital signs?

Q31. Disorder of sexual development (DSD)
Match the following signs occurring in association with DSD with the diagnosis.

Signs and symptoms	Diagnosis
a. Hypotonia, obesity	i. Fetal hydantoin
b. Anosmia	ii. Cornelia De lange
c. Retinitis pigmentosa	iii. Prader-Willi
d. Synophrys	iv. Bardet-Biedl
e. Hypoplasia of distal phalanges, growth failure	v. Kallman syndrome

Q32. Newborn rash

Parents are anxious about this generalized rash on a 2-day-old neonate.

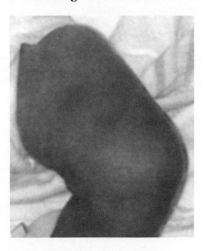

a.   What is the most likely diagnosis?

b.   What is the treatment and prognosis?

c.   What does the microscopic examination from the lesion reveal?

Q33. Given below is the X-ray of a 5-day-old male neonate who presented with abdominal distension.

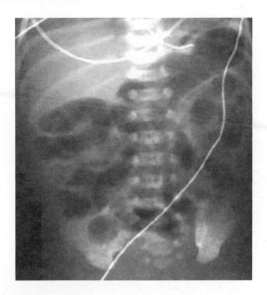

a.   What is the diagnosis?

b.   What are the predisposing factors?

c.   What is the diagnostic triad of this condition?

d.   Give details of classification used in accordance with severity of this disease.

Q34. Umbilical arterial line

After putting in a UA line, the right lower limb appears bluish-black.

a. What is the next step in management?
b. What is the level of the renal artery and celiac plexus in terms of vertebral levels?
c. How do you maintain a UA line?

Q35. A full term, male child develops jaundice on day 3 of life, (serum bilirubin 34 mg/dL) and is planned to undergo an exchange transfusion. Answer the following questions.

a. What is the complication likely to occur if left untreated?
b. Where is the anatomical location of the feared complication?
c. What are the long-term complications in this patient?
d. List 2 investigations you would perform prior to or soon after discharge.

Q36. A 15-days-old male newborn is noticed to have sweating and poor feeding of sudden onset. On examination, his HR is >240/min with signs of poor perfusion. There is no history maternal drug or alcohol abuse during pregnancy. There is no family history of similar problems.

a. What is the most likely diagnosis?
b. What is the immediate management?
c. Is DC shock the treatment of choice?

Q37. Given below is the photograph of scalp of a well term neonate.

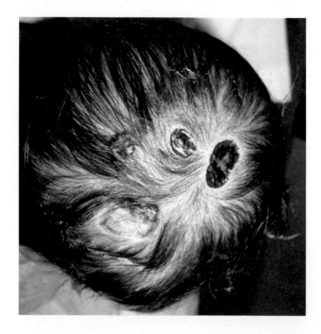

a. What is the most likely diagnosis?
b. What is the most common differential diagnosis of this condition?
c. List 3 conditions which can be associated with this condition

Q38. Given below is the image of a 30-week-old male neonate. He is diagnosed to have sepsis. He also has bleeding from the base of umbilical stump.

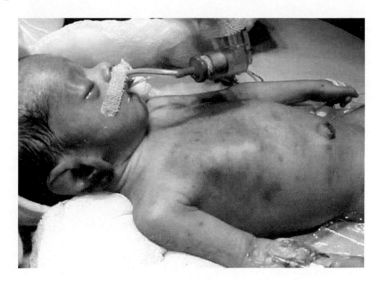

a. What is most likely diagnosis?
   He has had frequent episode of apnea and desaturation in past 2 hours.
b. List 2 most important investigations you will request in this neonate.
c. What is the most likely cause of his deterioration?

Q39. A 29-week-old neonate has had sudden increase in ventilatory requirement.

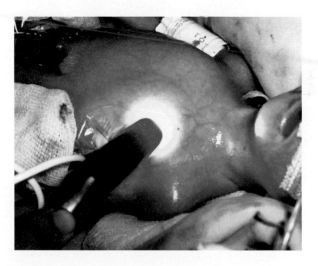

a. What is the test being performed?
b. What are the findings in a positive test performed above?
c. What is the diagnosis if the test is positive?

Q40. Given below is a picture of a 2-day-old term neonate.

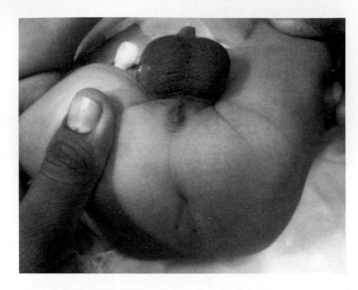

a. What is the diagnosis?
b. What is the definitive treatment?
c. What can be the long-term problem after the treatment?
d. List 4 associated malformations.

Q41. This is a term female infant was born via normal vaginal delivery.

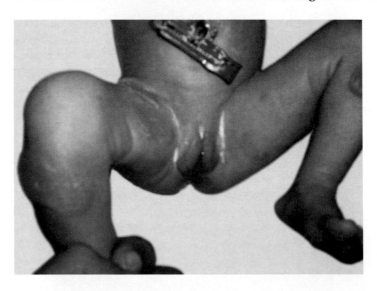

a. Describe the rash seen in picture above.
b. What is the most likely diagnosis?
c. What is the most common etiology/causative organism?
d. What is the treatment in this infant?

Q42. Given below is a term male neonate born via elective LSCS. Baby was born in poor condition and did not respond to any resuscitation.

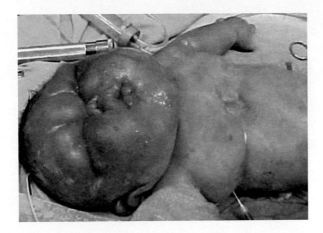

a. What is the most likely diagnosis?
b. List 1 pulmonary and 1 abdominal complication associated with this condition.
c. List 5 causes of the diagnosis including 2 where anemia is not an associated finding.

Q43. Given below is a photograph of a term male infant.

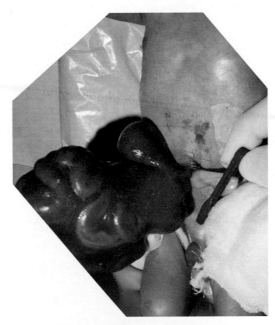

a. What is the most likely diagnosis?
b. What is the definitive treatment?
c. What is the most common complication seen later in childhood?

Q44. This term neonate is noted to have premature closure of sutures.

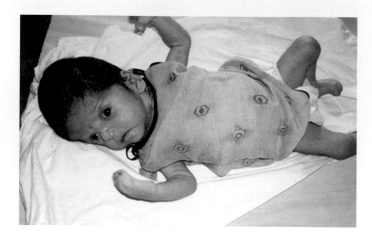

a. What is the most likely diagnosis?
b. List 2 clinical findings seen in this diagnosis.
c. What is the long-term problem?

Q45. This is photograph of a 1-month-old term infant.

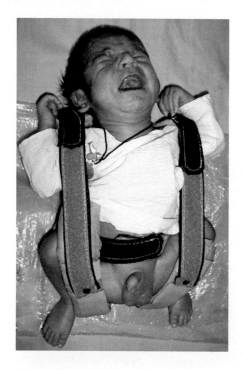

a. What is the equipment used on this infant?
b. What is the most likely problem with this infant?
c. What is the ideal age of the infant when this procedure is most successful?
d. What is the ideal duration of the total procedure?

Q46. This term neonate was born via normal vaginal delivery. He was initially covered with a tight glistening membrane.

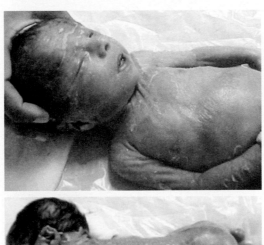

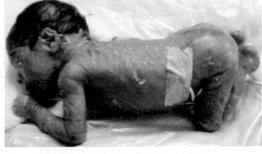

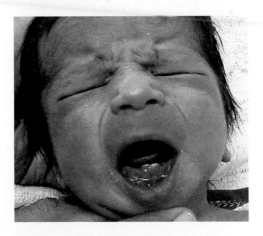

a. What is the most likely diagnosis?
b. List 2 possible immediate complications.
c. What is the immediate treatment?

Q47. Given below is the picture of a term female neonate.

a. What is the diagnosis?
b. List 2 condition associated with this diagnosis.
c. List 2 neonatal complication of this diagnosis.

Q48. A term newborn was noted to have audible cranial bruit. Given below is the MRA of this neonate.

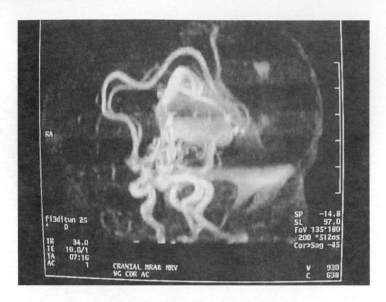

a. What is the most likely diagnosis?
b. List 2 most common complication associated with this condition.
c. Name 1 treatment option.

Q49. Given below is a picture of a 20-day-old term neonate.

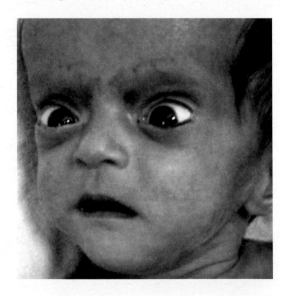

a. What is the sign seen in this photo?
b. What is the pathophysiology of this sign?
c. What is the most likely cause of this sign?

Q50. An 8-month-old infant presented in paediatric OPD with severe seborrheic dermatitis and bilateral otitis media. There is history of recurrent fever and weight loss over past 2 months. On examination, he is noted to have axillary lymphadenopathy and hepatosplenomegaly. Given below is the X-ray of this infant.

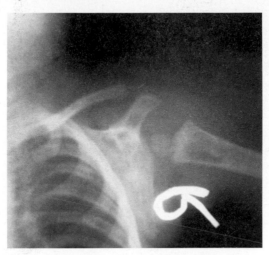

a. What is the finding seen on the chest X-ray?
b. What is the most likely diagnosis?
c. What is the treatment in this patient?

Q51. Given below is the X-ray of term neonate who was born via elective LSCS.

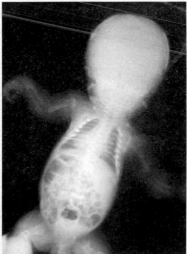

a. List 3 findings seen on X-ray.
b. What is the most likely diagnosis?
c. What are the clinical findings likely to be seen in this neonate?

Q52. A male newborn was born at 28 week gestation. He is now 4 weeks old and has needed 4 packed red cell transfusions. His current Hb is 6.8 mg/dL with low reticulocyte count. He is on full enteral feeds and iron (4 mg/kg/day) for past 10 days.

a. What is the most likely diagnosis?
b. What medication could have decreased the need for frequent blood transfusions in this neonate?
c. Give one non-hematological advantage of this medication.

Q53. A term neonate is noted to have petechiae and purpura all over the body on day 2 of life. His platelet counts are noted to be 60,000/mm³. Mother is a primigravida and known case of SLE. Her platelet counts are 70,000/mm³.

a. What is the most likely diagnosis in this newborn?
b. Enlist 2 generally accepted criteria for platelet transfusion in case of neonatal thrombocytopenia.
c. How do you define neonatal thrombocytopenia?
d. What is the treatment?

Q54. A 3 kg term ventilated neonate is nil by mouth. He is on 10% dextrose at rate of 9 mL/hr.

a. What is formula for calculating glucose infusion rate (GIR)?
b. Calculate the GIR for this baby.
c. What is the minimum GIR requirement of a neonate?

Q55. A 30-week female infant is about to be delivered via emergency LSCS in view of severe oilgohydramnios. The serial scans since 20 weeks have shown oligohydramnios.

a. Enlist 2 most common causes of oilgohydramnios.
b. Give 1 serious complication which might be seen on delivery of this neonate.

ANSWERS

A 1:

a. Colostomy
b. Anorectal malformation
   Artesia-Anal
   Atresia-Colon
   Hirschsprung's diseases.
c. Skin excoriation
   Prolapse of stoma
   Bleeding (chronic blood loss)
   Leakage
   Blockade.
d. Colostomy care/ stoma care
   Hydration of site-paraffin, etc.
   Care of surrounding skin.

A 2:

a. 5
b. 4
c. 5
d. 2

A 3:

a. Transillumination
b. Positive-transillumination, free gas in the abdomen
c. Suggestive of intestinal perforation
d. NBM, Surgical intervention
e. Chest- to rule out pneumothorax
f. Identification of veins.

A 4:

a. Colloidan baby
b. Incidence 1 in 600,000
c. Congenital ichthyosiform erythrodema
   Self-healing collodion baby
   Keratinization disorders ichthyosis vulgaris and trichothiodystrophy
   Other syndromes/disorder like Sjögren-Larsson syndrome, Netherton
   syndrome, Gaucher disease type 2, congenital hypothyroidism, Conradi
   syndrome, Dorfman-Chanarin syndrome, ketoadipiaciduria, koraxitrachitic
   syndrome, ichthyosis variegata and palmoplantar keratoderma with
   anogenital leukokeratosis.
d. Autosomal recessive
e. Immediate complications
   Cutaneous infection
   Aspiration pneumonia
   Hypothermia

Hypernatremic dehydration
Long term complications
Overheating:
Eye problems:
Constriction bands
Hair loss:
f. Immediate treatment
Admission in NICU
Prevention of dehydration and heat loss-ambient humidity/incubator/emmolients
Prevention of infections
Symptomatic relief
- Moisturizers
- Prevention of overheating
- Eye drops (to prevent the eyes from becoming dried out)
- Systemic retinoids
Psychological therapy

A 5:

1a Non Protein Calories = Lipid Calories + Dextrose calories

$$= \text{Gram of lipid} \times 10 + \text{Gram of Dextrose} \times 3.5$$
$$= (2 \times 1.2) \times 10 + (6 \times 1.44 \times 1.2) \times 3.5$$
$$= 24+36.28 = 60.28$$

Nitrogen

$$= \text{Protein} \times 0.16$$
$$= 3 \times 1.2 \times 0.16$$
$$= 0.576$$

$$\frac{\text{NPC}}{\text{N}} = \frac{60.28}{0.3576} = 104.5$$

1b Range of 100-150 NPC/N is desirable for utilisation of protein.

2a $\dfrac{\text{Protein} \times \text{Weight}}{\% \text{ of protein solution} \times 24}$

$$\frac{3 \times 102}{0.1 \times 24} = \frac{3.6}{2.4} = 1.5 \text{ mL/hr}$$

b. $\dfrac{\text{Lipid} \times \text{Weight}}{\% \text{ of lipid solution} \times 24}$

$$\frac{2 \times 1.2}{0.2 \times 24} = 0.5 \text{ mL/hr}$$

c. $\dfrac{\text{Glucose} \times \text{Weight}}{\% \text{ of glucose solution} \times 24}$

$$\frac{6 \times 1.44 \times 1.2}{0.5 \times 24} = 0.864 \text{ mL/hr}$$

3. Total Calories
= Protein calories + Lipid calories + Glucose calories
= $(3 \times 1.2 \times 4) + (2 \times 1.2 \times 10) + (6 \times 1.44 \times 1.2 \times 3.5)$
= 14.4 + 24 + 36.288
= 74.7 calories/kg/day or 62 calories/day
3b   90-110.

A 6:

1-b 2-c 3-d 4e 5a

A 7:

a. Exomphalos major/omphalocele.
b.   i. Transport supine with the hernia suspended by a string
    ii. Cover the omphalocele with a waterproof covering
    iii. Provide additional fluids
    iv. Maintain body temperature
     v. Place an orogastric tube.
c. Beckwith Weidemann syndrome, cardiac anomalies e.g. TOF and ASD, chromosomal abnormalities e.g. various trisomies, genitourinary anomalies, diaphragmatic hernia.
d. Surgical correction (usually non-urgent, staged closure).

A 8:

a. HIE/perinatal asphyxia:
   —   Sepsis/meningitis.
   —   Inborn error of metabolism/pyridoxine deficiency.
   —   Birth trauma.
b.   i. Management of the airway, breathing and circulation.
    ii. Do the blood sugar; if < 40 mg%, give a bolus of 2 mL/kg of D 10%; If > 40 mg% proceed to next step.
    iii. Take sample for serum calcium; give IV calcium gluconate 2 mL/kg 1:1 diluted.
    iv. Give IV Phenobarbitone in a dose of 20 mg/kg as a slow iv injection.
     v. Repeat IV Phenobarbitone in a dose of 5–10 mg/kg up to maximum total dose of 40 mg/kg.
    vi. Phenytoin the usual second-line agent, is given as an initial loading dose of 20 mg/kg.
   vii. Benzodiazepines (e.g. Lorazepam, diazepam, and midazolam). For neonatal seizures that remain refractory to these measures, benzodiazepines may add further benefit.

A 9:

a.   i. Ability to maintain temperature in an open crib.
    ii. Ability to take all feedings by bottle or breast without respiratory compromise.
    iii. No apnea or bradycardia for 5 days.
    iv. Steady weight gain.
b.   i. Yes

    ii. Yes

    iii. Yes

A 10:

a. HBeAg and anti HBe Ag.

b. Anti HBs Ag +ve.

c. Husband to get his HBs Ag status checked and to use barrier contraception during sexual intercourse.

d. Give first dose of hepatitis B vaccine and HBIG concurrently at different sites within 12 hours of birth followed by hepatitis B vaccine at 1 and 6 months.

A 11:

a. It implies in utero infection and possibly a rapidly progressive disease.

b. By repeating the sample. A diagnosis of HIV infection can be made with 2 positive virologic test results obtained from different blood samples.

c.   i. Nucleoside/nucleotide reverse transcriptase inhibitors (NRTIS). Zidovudine, didanosine, tenofovir, stavudine, abacavir.

    ii. Non-nucleoside reverse transcriptase inhibitors (NNRTIS). Nevirapine, Efavirenz.

    iii. Protease inhibitors: Nelfinavir, amprenavir, atazanavir, darunavir, fosamprenavir, indinavir, lopinavir/ritonavir, saquinavir.

A 12:

a. Vitamin K deficiency (classical).

b. Administration of total parentral alimentation.
Administration of parenteral antibiotics.
Prematurity.

c. Parentral administration of vitamin K to all newborns at the time of birth.

d. 1 mg IV or IM vitamin K.

A 13:

a. CHARGE:

C	-	Coloboma of the eye, central nervous system anomalies
H	-	Heart defects
A	-	Atresia of the choanae
R	-	Retardation of growth and/or development
G	-	Genital and/or urinary defects (hypogonadism)
E	-	Ear anomalies and/or deafness.

b. Heart defects
Retardation of growth and/or development.

c. ECHO

d. Transnasal repair.

A 14:

a. Arm is held in adduction, elbow extended, internally rotated, forearm pronated and wrist flexed (Waiters tip position).

b. Erb palsy.

c. Injury to upper nerve roots of brachial plexus – C5 + C6 ± C7.
d. Phrenic nerve involvement—Ipsilateral diaphragmatic paralysis.

A 15:

Type of chorion and amnion	Timing of division of egg
a. Monochorionic, monoamniotic	7–14 days
b. Monochorionic, diamniotic	3–7 days
c. Dichorionic, diamniotic	0–3 days
d. Conjoint twins	>14 days

A 16:
a. Periventricular calcifications.
   Ventricular dilatation.
b. Congenital CMV infection.
c. Hepatosplenomegaly.
   Sensorineural hearing loss.
   Chorioretinitis.
   Thrombocytopenia.
   Encephalopathy.

A 17:
a. Uncompensated respiratory acidosis.
b. Increase the rate.
c. Size 2.5.

A 18:
a. Partially compensated respiratory alkalosis with hyperoxia.
b. Decrease PIP.
c. Periventricular leucomalacia/intraventricular hemorrhage.

A 19:

a. $$\frac{(\text{Blood volume/kg} \times \text{weight in kg}) \times (\text{Observed-desired hematocrit})}{\text{Observed hematocrit}}$$

b. $$= \frac{80 \times 2 \times (80 - 50)}{80} = 60 \text{ mL}$$

c. Hypoglycemia
   Thrombotic episode
   Congestive cardiac failure
   NEC
   Thrombocytopenia
   DIC.

A 20:
a. Hypoxemia.
b. Increase PEEP.
c. HFOV.

A 21:

a. Klumpke palsy.
b. Injury to lower nerve roots of brachial plexus – C7 + C8 + T1.
c. Horner syndrome.

A 22:

a. Uncompensated metabolic acidosis.
b. Shock.
c. IV Bolus of normal saline 10 mL/kg over 20–30 minutes.

A 23:

a. Dopamine.
   Dobutamine.
b. Disconnect from ventilator transiently at the time of measurement.
c. 5 to 8 mm Hg.
d. Intrathoracic inferior vena cava.
e. Maintaining CVP at 5 to 8 mm Hg with volume infusions is associated with improved cardiac output. If CVP exceeds 5 to 8 mm Hg, additional volume will usually not be helpful.

A 24:

a. 4-6 cm H_2O.
b. Pneumothorax.
   Nasal septum injury.
   Gastric distention.
   Decrease venous return secondary to increased intrathoracic pressure.
c. Congenital diaphragmatic hernia.
   Upper airway malformations like—Choanal atresia, cleft palate.

A 25:

a. Persistent pulmonary hypertension of newborn.
b. Nitric oxide.
c. ECMO.
d. Sildenafil, adenosine, magnesium sulfate, calcium channel blockers, inhaled prostacyclin, inhaled ethyl nitrite, and inhaled or intravenous tolazoline.

A 26:

a. Polycythemia.
b. Venous hematocrit of over 65%
   Venous hematocrit of over 64% or more at 2 hours of age
   An umbilical venous or arterial hematocrit of over 63% or more.
c. Partial exchange transfusion.

A 27:

a. Congenital clubfoot or talipes equinocavovarus with metatarsal adduction.
b. First-degree relative suffering from the same condition:
   Oligohydramnios
   Neurologic dysfunction of the feet, e.g. spina bifida.

c. Components:
   - Equinus position of foot
   - Cavus position of foot
   - Varus position of foot
   - Forefoot adduction (occasionally).
d. Physical therapy and splinting. Manipulation and application of tapes, plaster or fiberglass casts.
   Serial casting followed by heel cord tenotomy (Ponseti method of management).

A 28:

a. Pan-hypopituitarism.
b. •Cortisol and growth hormone
   - Magnetic resonance imaging to visualize the hypothalamus and pituitary.

A 29:

a. Pendred syndrome.
b. Autosomal recessive.
c. Thyroid hormone synthetic defects.
d. Normal thyroid seen.

A 30:

a. Hypoxic-ischemic encephalopathy.
b. Stage 2 (moderate)—Sarnat and sarnat staging.
c. 36 weeks.
d. 80% normal; abnormal if symptoms more than 5 to 7 days.
e. Improvement in heart rate followed by improvement in color followed by improvement in tone.

A 31:

Signs and symptoms	Diagnosis
a. Hypotonia, obesity	• Prader-Willi
b. Anosmia	• Kallman syndrome
c. Retinitis pigmentosa	• Bardet-Biedl
d. Synophrys	• Cornelia De lange
e. Hypoplasia of distal phalanges, growth failure	• Fetal hydantoin

A 32:

a. Erythema toxicum neonatorum.
b. Self limiting—no treatment required.
c. Inflammatory cells with >90% eosinophils.

A 33:

a. The diagnosis is NEC.
b. Sepsis, prematurity, hypoxic or hemodynamic insult, etc.
c. Acidosis, hyponatremia, thrombocytopenia.

d. Bell staging criteria.
    Stage I (suspect): Clinical signs and symptoms, nondiagnostic radiographs.
    Stage II (definite) : Clinical signs and symptoms, pneumatosis intestinalis on radiograph:
    a   Mildly ill
    b. Moderately ill with systemic toxicity.
    Stage III (Advanced): Clinical signs and symptoms, pneumatosis intestinalis on radiograph, and critically ill:
    a. Impending intestinal perforation
    b. Proven intestinal perforation.

A 34:

a. Remove the UAC.
b. L1 and T12.
c. Continuous heparinised saline infusion.

A 35:

a. Kernicterus/bilirubin encephalopathy.
b. Globus pallidus, dentate nucleus, cerebellar vermis, cochlear nuclei.
c. Choreoathetoid cerebral palsy, dystonic/dyskinetic CP, sensorineural deafness.
d. Audiometry testing.
    MRI

A 36:

a. Supraventricular tachycardia.
b. Vagal stimulation followed by IV adenosine.
c. No.

A 37:

a. Aplasia cutis congenita
    Multiple, small, non-inflammatory, well-demarcated, oval ulcers.
b. Traumatic skin injury from monitoring devices, e.g. scalp electrodes.
c. Opitz syndrome:
    Adams-Oliver syndrome
    Oculocerebrocutaneous syndrome
    Johanson-Blizzard syndrome
    4p(-) microdeletion syndromes
    X-p22 microdeletion syndromes
    trisomy 13–15
    Chromosome 16–18 defects.

A 38:

a. DIC.
b. Clotting profile, cranial ultrasound.
c. IVH.

A 39:

a. Transillumination.
b. Hyperlucency in the affected area.
c. Pneumothorax.

A 40:

a. Imperforate anus.
b. Low—Surgical dilatation.
   High—Initial colostomy with a definitive repair at a later stage.
c. Rectal inertia/constipation.
d. *Genitourinary:* Vesicoureteric reflux, renal agenesis, renal dysplasia, ureteral duplication, cryptorchidism, hypospadias, bicornuate uterus, vaginal septums.
   Vertebral: Spinal dysraphism, tethered chord, presacral masses, meningocele, lipoma, dermoid, teratoma.
   Cardiovascular: Tetralogy of fallot, ventricular septal defect, transposition of the great vessels, hypoplastic left heart syndrome.
   Gastrointestinal: Tracheoesophageal fistula, duodenal atresia, malrotation, Hirschsprung disease.

A 41:

a. Widespread honey colored bullae.
b. Impetigo.
c. *Staph. aureus.*
d. Cloxacillin (antistaphylococcal antibiotics).

A 42:

a. Hydrops fetalis.
b. Pleural effusion and ascites.
c. Associated with anemia:
   i. Haemolytic disease of newborn
   ii. Chronic twin to twin transfusion
   iii. Feto maternal haemorrhage
   iv. Parvo virus B_{19}.

   Anemia is not an associated finding:
   i. Cardiac failure, e.g. in SVT
   ii. Congenital nephrotic syndrome
   iii. Chromosomal abnormalities, e.g. Turners.

A 43:

a. Gastroschisis.
b. Surgery: Staged or primary closure.
c. Short bowel syndrome.

A 44:

a. Apert syndrome.
b. Asymmetry of head shape—Premature fusion of multiple sutures.
   Syndactyly of the 2nd, 3rd, and 4th fingers.
   Congenital cataract.
c. Progressive calcification and fusion of the bones of the hands, feet, and cervical spine.

A 45:

a. Pavlik harness.
b. Developmental dysplasia of the hip.
c. 1–6 months—success rate >95%.
d. 6 weeks.

A 46:

a. Collodion baby.
b. Skin infection/sepsis
   Dehydration
   Hypothermia.
c. Intensive care in a humidified environment
   Regular application of oil
   High fluid intake with careful electrolyte monitoring
   Early recognition and treatment of sepsis.

A 47:

a. Natal teeth.
b. Cleft palate
   Pierre-Robin syndrome
   Ellis-van creveld syndrome
   Hallermann-Streiff syndrome
   Pachyonychia congenita.
c. Pain and refusal to feed
   Maternal discomfort because of nipple abrasion
   Detachment and aspiration of the tooth
   Antenatal laceration or amputation of tongue (Riga-Fede disease).

A 48:

a. Vein of Galen malformation.
b. Hydrocephalous
   High output cardiac failure.
c. Coil embolisation.

A 49:

a. Sun setting sign—the eyes deviate downward.
b. Impingement of the dilated suprapineal recess on the tectum.
c. Hydrocephalous.

A 50:

a. Multiple osteolytic bone lesions.
b. Langerhans cell histiocytosis type 1.
c. Chemotherapy in view of multisystem involvement.

A 51:

a. Multiple fractures.
   Relative large head.
   Flaring of thoracic cage.
   Short extremities.

b. Osteogenesis imperfecta.
c. Blue sclera
   Hearing loss
   Orthopedic abnormalities

   CVS abnormalities (mitral valve prolapse).

A 52:

a. Late anemia of prematurity.
b. Erythropoietin.
c. Decrease incidence of bronchopulmonary dysplasia.

A 53:

a. Autoimmune thrombocytopenia (automaternal ITP).
b. Platelet count <20,000
   Bleeding neonate.
c. Platelet count <150,000.
d. Platelet transfusion
   IVIG
   Steroid—Prednisolone 2 mg/kg/day.

A 54:

a. $\text{GIR in mg/kg/min} = \dfrac{\text{Dextrose concentration} \times \text{ml/kg/day}}{144}$

b. $\dfrac{10 \times 72}{144} = 5 \text{ mg/kg/min}$

c. 4 mg/kg/min.

A 55:

a. Amniotic fluid leak, e.g. ROM
   Renal dysgenesis or agenesis.
b. Pulmonary hypoplasia
   Arthrogryposis/joint deformity.

QUESTIONS

Q1.

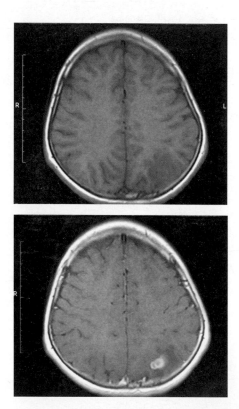

a. What is the radiological finding?
b. What is the diagnosis?
c. Enlist 2 commonest clinical conditions leading into above abnormalities.
d. What is cause of difference in radiological finding between 2 images?

Q2.

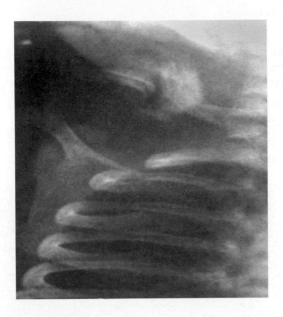

a. What is the diagnosis?
b. What is the commonest cause of abnormality in neonates and older child?
c. What is the treatment?

Q3. A 12-year-old boy presented with first episode of nonfebrile left focal seizures.

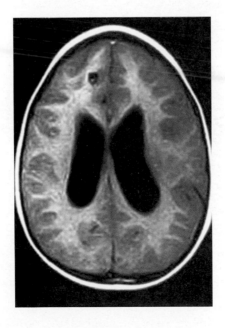

a. What is the most likely diagnosis?
b. What is the etiology?
c. What is the treatment?

Q4. A 12-year-old boy presented with history of fever, headache and generalized tonic clonic seizures. His MRI shows hypertense lesion in the right temporal lobe.

a. What is the most likely diagnosis?
b. How can you confirm the diagnosis?
c. What is the drug of choice?

Q5. Answer following questions based on X-ray seen.

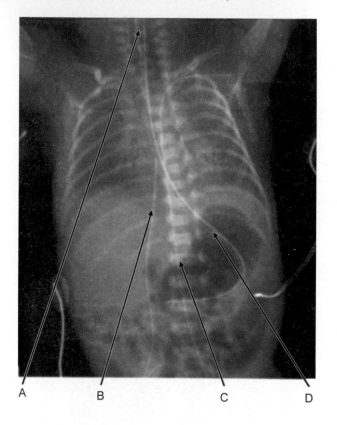

A   B   C   D

a. What are A, B, C and D?
b. What is the ideal position of placement of A, B, C and D on X-ray?
c. Which of the above is incorrectly placed?

Q6. A 10-year-old girl was admitted in PICU for acute gastroenteritis with severe dehydration. 24 hours after the admission she had an episode of generalized seizures. On examination, her Glasgow coma scale score is 7,

heart rate 60/min, respirations are irregular and blood pressure is normal. Review the CT given below and answer the questions.

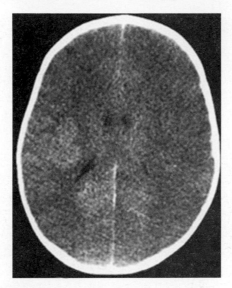

a. What are your findings on the CT scan?
b. What is the immediate management after the "ABC"?
c. What is the most common electrolyte disturbance which can be the cause of above problem in this patient?

Q7. Given below is the chest X-ray of a 6-week-old male infant. The infant has been having persistent tachypnea since birth. He has been treated with multiple courses of antibiotics for presumed pneumonia. Study the X-ray and answer the questions.

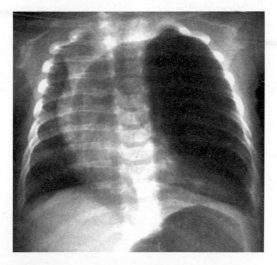

a. List 3 positive findings on chest X-ray.
b. What is the diagnosis in this X-ray?
c. What is the most common site of involvement in the above diagnosis?

Q8. Given below is the X-ray of a term male infant who presented with abdominal distention.

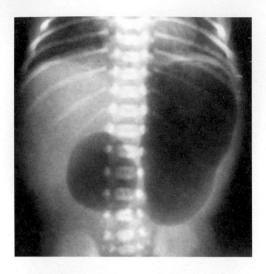

a. Name the abnormality seen.
b. What is the likely diagnosis?
c. What is the commonest chromosomal aberration associated with this abnormality?
d. What is the commonest upper gastrointestinal abnormality associated with this abnormality?

Q9. A term female newborn was noted to have significant respiratory distress soon after birth. Study the X-ray and answer the questions.

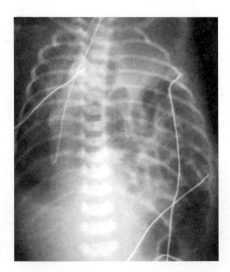

a. Describe the X-ray findings.
b. What is the diagnosis?

   c. List 2 precautions to be taken during resuscitation to avoid any further deterioration in the clinical condition.

   d. What other anomalies can be associated with this condition?

Q10. Given below is an X-ray of a 24-hour-old neonate.

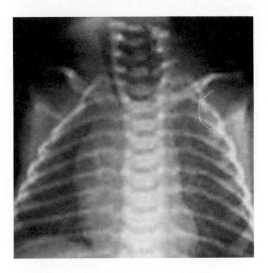

   a. What is the most likely diagnosis?

   b. Which is the most common subtype?

   c. Give one common association with this condition.

Q11. Given below is X-ray of a 12-year-old seen by dentist with multiple dental abnormalities. This child has a history of delayed closure of fontanel and droopy shoulders.

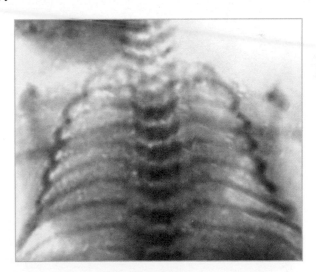

   a. What is the abnormality on the X-ray?

   b. What is the likely diagnosis?

c. List 3 abnormalities which are commonly seen with this diagnosis.

d. What is the clinical sign supporting the pathology seen in the X-ray above?

Q12. Given below is the HIDA scan of a 2 months old 6 hours post dye injection.

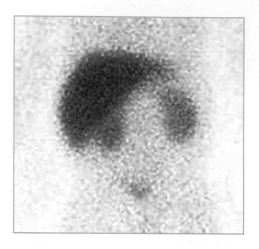

a. What are the findings on the scan?

b. What is the most likely diagnosis?

c. Which dye is used in this scan?

d. List any 6 supplementary medications required for this infant (including the dosing of any 4).

Q13. A 15-month-old child was brought to pediatric emergency room with history of sudden onset of cough and choking. While coming to the Hospital he became asymptomatic. A chest X-ray performed is given below.

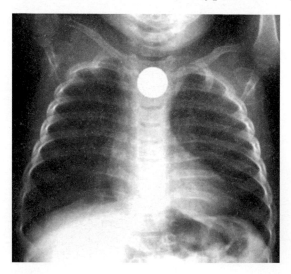

a. What is the diagnosis?

b. List 2 possible complications.

c. What is the definitive treatment for this child?
   This child has a sudden cardiorespiratory deterioration while in emergency.
d. What is the next step in management?

Q14. This 12-year-old was intubated on arrival at emergency room following a road accident. Her intubation was difficult needing multiple attempts. The X-ray provided below was performed soon after admission.

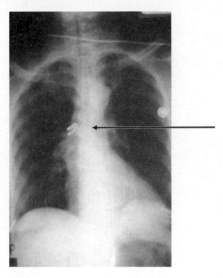

a. What is foreign body pointed in the X-ray?
b. Where is the location of this foreign body?
c. How would you remove the foreign body?

Q15. A 11-month-old male infant presented to pediatric OPD with high-grade fever and labored breathing. On auscultation, breath sounds are barely audible on right side. The X-ray performed is shown below.

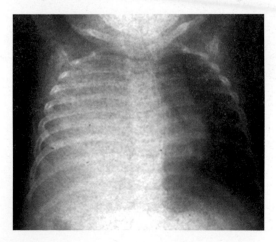

a. List 3 positive findings on chest X-ray.
b. What is the likely diagnosis?

Q16. This is an X-ray of the abdomen in a 12-year-old girl who was brought to the pediatric OPD with chief complaint of recurrent abdominal pain. She has been bedridden since age of 7 years due to paraplegia following transverse myelitis.

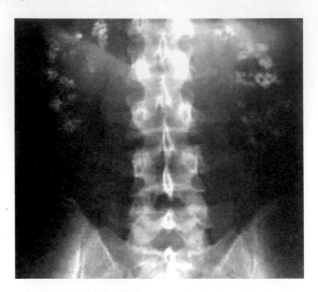

a. What abnormality can be seen on the plain abdominal film?
b. What is the diagnosis?
c. What are the definitive treatment options? (List any 2)
d. List 4 causes of this radiological finding.

Q17. A 3-year-old presented with an abdominal mass and hypertension. On investigation, she was noted to have microscopic hematuria. The CT scan performed show a large nonoccupying more than 70% of the abdomen.

a. What is the likely diagnosis?
b. List 2 syndromes associated with this condition.

Q18. A 5-year-old is diagnosed to have unilateral Wilms tumour. As a part of further investigation and staging of the disease, a CT scan of chest was performed.

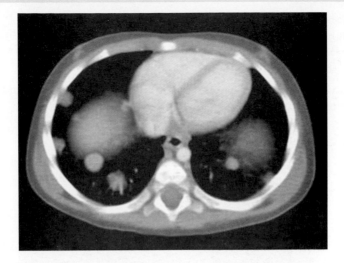

a. What is the finding on the CT scan?
b. What is the staging of his disease?
c. What other investigation will guide the treatment?
d. What is the treatment?

Q19. Given below is the CT scan of a 2-month-old. This child was born at term and had a stormy neonatal course. He was diagnosed to have neonatal sepsis and seizures on day 3 of life and was treated with antibiotics for 7 days.

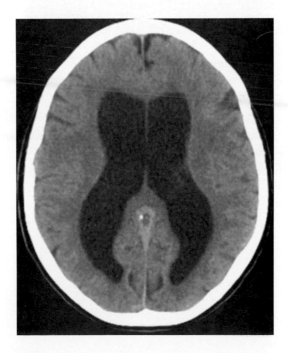

a. What is the radiological diagnosis?
b. What is the most likely cause in this infant?
c. How do you calculate VP ratio?
d. What is the medical management of the condition?

Q20. A 8-year-old child presents to pediatric OPD with history of drooling of saliva and high-grade fever.

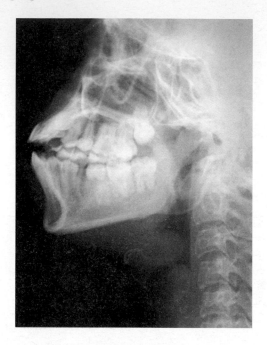

a. What is the most likely diagnosis?
b. What is the commonest organism causing this problem?
c. What is the treatment after stabilization of the child?

Q21. An incidental finding was noted on reviewing the abdominal CT of a 12-year-old male for abdominal pain. The finding was later confirmed on history and physical examination.

a. What is the radiological finding in the inguinal section of abdominal CT given below?

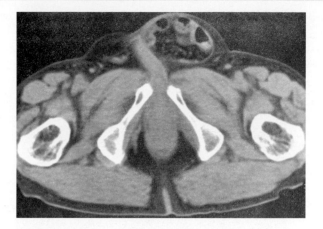

b. What is the diagnosis?
c. What is the treatment?

Q22. Given below is an X-ray of a 3-year-old female child with frontal bossing, bowing of legs and a large abdomen.

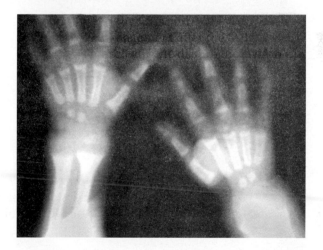

a. What are the findings seen on the X-ray?
b. What is the most likely diagnosis?
c. Enlist 3 common skeletal deformities seen in association with this disease.
d. What is the biochemical abnormality seen in this disease?

Q23. Identify the structures shown in cranial USG shown below.

a.

b.

c.

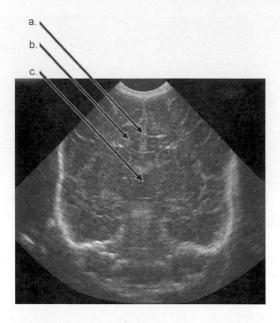

Q24. A 28-week-old male infant is admitted to NICU. Given below is the cranial USG of this neonate at 48 hour age.

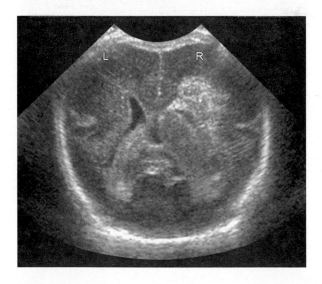

a. What are the cranial ultrasound findings?
b. What is the complete diagnosis?
c. How do you stage the disease based on cranial USG?

Q25. Given below is the cranial USG of a 27-week-old female neonate.

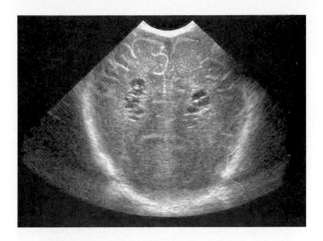

a. What are the cranial ultrasound findings?
b. What is the diagnosis?
c. What is the most likely cause of the diagnosis?

Q26. Given below is the X-ray of 14-year-old male following a road traffic accident.

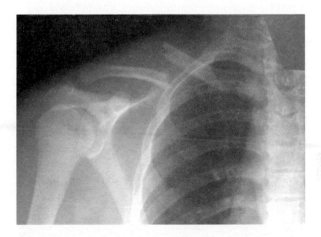

a. What is the abnormality seen on the X-ray above?
b. List 1 possible complication.

Q27. A 32-week-old male infant is born via spontaneous vaginal delivery. He was born in good condition and did not require any resuscitation. Mother had no antenatal concerns and did not receive any medications

prior to delivery. Baby developed respiratory distress soon after birth and was intubated and ventilated.

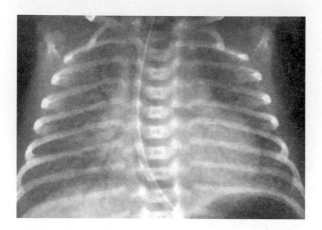

a. What is the most likely diagnosis on chest X-ray?
b. List two most important findings suggesting the diagnosis on chest X-ray.
c. What maternal intervention could have decreased the incidence of the likely diagnosis?

Q28. A 35-week-old female is born via elective LSCS. She cried soon after birth and did not require any resuscitation. She is born to a primigravida mother, who had no risk factors for sepsis. She developed tachypnea soon after birth with mild to moderate subcostal recessions.

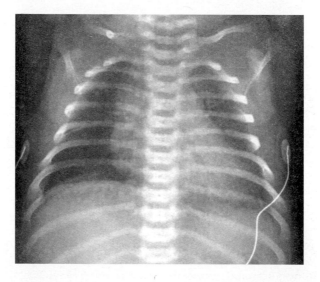

a. List two positive findings on chest X-ray.
b. What is the likely diagnosis?
c. What is prognosis?
d. Is there a role of diuretics in this condition?

Q29. A 4 kg 42-week-old male infant was born at home. The pregnancy was unbooked. No other antenatal details are available. The newborn is admitted to NICU with severe respiratory distress. His saturation is 72% in free flow oxygen. An IV cannula is sited and his blood sugar is 28 mg. His capillary blood gas shows.

pH	7.01
pCO_2	78
pO_2	30
HCO_3^-	12

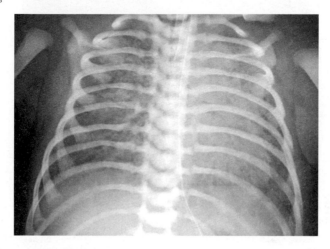

a. List the positive findings on chest X-ray.
b. What is the likely diagnosis?
c. List 3 most important steps in management of this neonate.

Q30. A preterm ventilated baby had a hemodynamic compromise of sudden onset. The chest X-ray is given below.

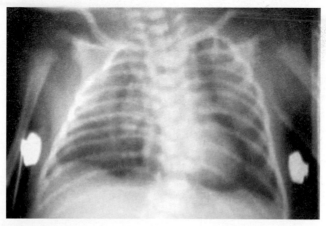

a. What is the diagnosis?
b. List two bedside procedures, which could have helped in confirming the diagnosis before performing the X-ray.

c. What is the definitive treatment in this neonate?
d. What is the treatment option if the infant was asymptomatic?

Q31. This term neonate was born via normal vaginal delivery. He was noted to have significant respiratory distress soon after birth.

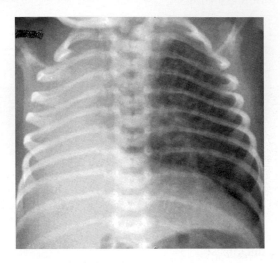

a. What are the findings on the chest X-ray?
b. What is the most likely diagnosis?
c. Give one congenital abnormality, which can be associated with this condition.

Q32. This 12-year-old presents in pediatric OPD with respiratory distress of one day duration. He was reviewed in the OPD two days back with complaint of cough and cold and was diagnosed to have viral URI.

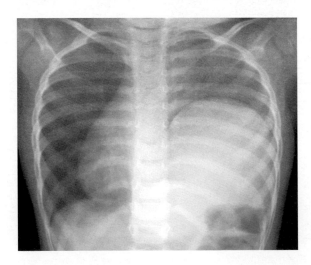

a. What is the most likely diagnosis?
b. How would you confirm the diagnosis?

Q33. Given below is the X-ray of a 12-year-old female who presented to pediatric OPD with complaint of back pain.

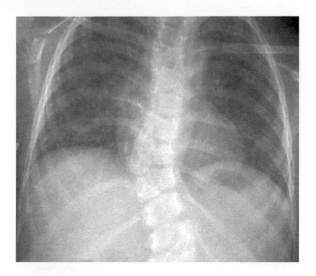

a. What is the diagnosis?
b. What extent of above disease causes cardiopulmonary compromise?
c. What is the definitive indication of surgery in this diagnosis?
d. List four conditions which can be associated with this diagnosis.

Q34. Identify the cardiac disease on the basis of the chest X-ray in this neonate.

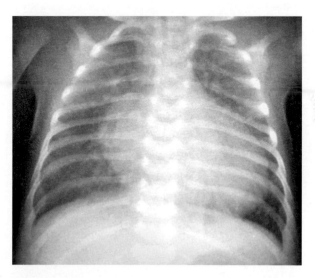

a. What is the diagnosis?
b. What is the name given to this typical chest X-ray presentation?
c. Name the drug used in this neonate soon after birth.
   The infant's condition fails to improve despite of above drug.

d. Name the procedure which can be performed prior to the definitive surgery.
e. Name the surgical procedures used to correct this anomaly and what age is this procedure performed?

Q35. Identify the cardiac disease on the basis of the chest X-ray.

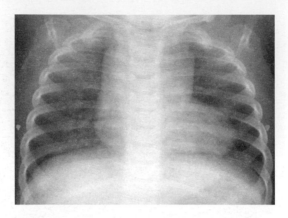

a. What is the diagnosis?
b. What is the name given to this typical chest X-ray presentation?
c. What are findings on cardiac examination?
d. List two most common neurological complications associated with the above diagnosis.

Q36. Identify the cardiac disease on the basis of the chest X-ray.

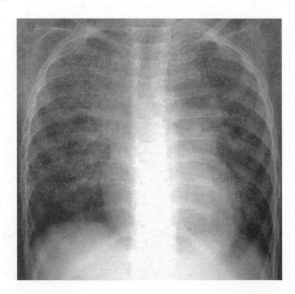

a. What is the diagnosis?
b. What is the name given to this typical chest X-ray presentation?
c. What is the clinical presentation of the infant with this diagnosis?

ANSWERS

A 1:

a. Hypointense lesion in posterior occipital lobe
b. Ring enhancing lesion
c. Inflammatory granuloma
d. TBM, neurocysticercosis
e. Image B is post contrast.

A 2:

a. Clavicular fracture with callus formation
b. Neonate—birth trauma
   Older child—direct trauma to the clavicle
c. Conservative in most cases rarely needing surgical correction.

A 3:

a. Neurocysticercosis (with mild ventricular dilatation).
b. *Taenia solium* or pork tape worm.
c. Albendazole (15 mg/kg/day, BID) for 28 days with steroids for 2–3 days before and immediately after initiating therapy.
   Anticonvulsant—carbamazepine or phenytoin.

A 4:

a. HSV encephalitis.
b. CSF viral studies for HSV-PCR.
c. IV Acyclovir (5–10 mg/kg or 250 mg/m^2 every 8 hour).

A 5:

a. A-Endotracheal tube.
   B and C-Umbilical venous cannula and umbilical arterial cannula.
   D-Nasogastric tube.
b. A-Endotracheal tube: T2-T3.
   B and C-Umbilical venous cannula—Just above the diaphragm and umbilical arterial cannula, high:T7-T10; low: L2-L3.
   D-Nasogastric tube—In the stomach.
c. All of the above.

A 6:

a. Cerebral edema in view of loss distinctness of the sulci and gyri. Due to increased ICP, the cortex is compressed up against the skull. The space between the cortex and the skull is obliterated.
b. Hyperventilation, mannitol.
c. Hyponatremia.

A 7:

a. Hyperinflation of the left upper lobe.
   Paucity of vascular markings of the left upper lobe.
   Mediastinal shift to the right.

Atelectasis of the left lower lobe.
Flattening of the left hemidiaphragm.
b. Congenital lobar emphysema.
c. Left upper lobe.

A 8:

a. Double bubble appearance.
b. Duodenal atresia.
c. Down's syndrome.
d. Annular pancreas.

A 9:

a. There is a cystic mass (bowel loops) on the left side displacing the heart to the opposite side.
b. Congenital diaphragmatic hernia.
c. Place an OG/NG tube.
   Not to give IPPV via bag and mask.
d. Pulmonary hypoplasia/aplasia with congenital heart disease, Cantrell's pentalogy.

A 10:

a. Esophageal atresia.
b. Esophageal atresia with distal TEF (85%).
c. VATER/VACTREL.

A 11:

a. Absent clavicles.
b. Cleidocranial dysplasia.
c. i. Drooping shoulders.
    ii. Open fontanelles, prominent forehead, mild short stature—because of delayed ossification of the cranial bones with multiple ossification centers (wormian bones), and delayed ossification of pelvic bones.
    iii. Dental anomalies (numerous teeth abnormalities including delayed eruption of teeth).
d. Both shoulders can be approximated together anteriorly.

A 12:

a. No dye reaching the intestine.
b. Biliary atresia.
c. Iminodiacetic acid (Tc iminodiacetic) compound.
d. Aquasol A—10,000-15,000 IU/day.
   Oral α-tocopherol or TPGS 50–400 IU/day.
   25-hydroxycholecalciferol 3-5 μg/kg/day or D2 5,000–8,000 IU/day.
   Water-soluble derivative of menadione 2.5—5.0 mg every other day.
   Calcium, phosphate, or zinc supplementation.
   Choleretic bile acids and ursodeoxycholic acid, 15-20 mg/kg/day.
   Dietary formula or supplements containing medium-chain triglycerides.

A 13:

a. Esophageal foreign body.
b. Esophageal perforation.
   Oesophageal obstruction.
   Tracheal compression.
c. Endoscopy—diagnostic and therapeutic.
d. 5 abdominal thrust (Hemlich manouver) with the child sitting or lying down.

A 14:

a. Broken tooth.
b. Right main bronchus.
c. Rigid bronchoscopy.

A 15:

a. Diffuse homogenous opacity in entire right lung field.
   Mediastinal shift to left side.
   Obliterated right CP angle.
b. Right pleural effusion.

A 16:

a. Bilateral radiopacities seen in the X-rays—calcification of kidneys.
b. Nephrocalcinosis.
c. Shock wave lithotripsy
   Ureteroscopy.
   Percutaneous nephrolithotomy.
d. Drug—Frusemide therapy
   Medullary sponge kidney
   Hyperoxalemia
   Renal tubular acidosis
   Hypoparathyroidism
   Hypophosphatemic rickets
   Sarcoidosis
   Prolonged immobilization.

A 17:

a. Wilms' tumor.
b. WAGR syndrome is a contiguous gene deletion syndrome that consists of Wilms tumor, aniridia, genitourinary abnormalities
   Beckwith-Wiedemann syndrome
   Denys-Drash—Early onset renal failure with renal mesangial sclerosis, male pseudohermaphrodism, increased risk of Wilms tumor.

A 18:

a. Bilateral pulmonary metastases.
b. Stage IV.
c. Histopathology—Favorable/anaplastic.
d. Surgical extirpation, chemotherapy and radiotherapy.

For stage IV tumors with favorable histology, vincristine, actinomycin D, and doxorubicin are administered, and radiation therapy is also administered to all the sites of known disease, particularly the lungs.

For tumors with unfavorable histology, vincristine, actinomycin D, doxorubicin, and cyclophosphamide are administered, and radiation therapy is also administered to all the known sites of disease.

A 19:

a. Hydrocephalous.
b. Neonatal meningitis.
c. Divide the maximum ventricular measurement by maximum parenchymal measurement at the level of third ventricle.
d. Acetazolamide and furosemide to decrease secretion by choroid plexus.

A 20:

a. Epiglottitis.
b. *H. influenzae.*
c. IV antibiotics—Ceftriaxone, cefotaxime, or a combination of ampicillin and sulbactam.

A 21:

a. Gas—containing bowel loops as well as mesenteric fat and vessels in the left inguinal canal.
b. Inguinal hernia.
c. Surgical repair.

A 22:

a. Fraying of metaphysis
   Cupping of distal end of radius and ulna
   Widening of distal end of metaphysis
   Generalized rarefaction.
b. Rickets
c. *Head:* Craniotabes, frontal bossing, delayed fontanelle closure, craniosynostosis
   Back: Scoliosis, kyphosis, lordosis
   Chest: Rachitic rosary, harrison groove
   Extremities: Enlargement of wrists and ankles
      Valgus or varus deformities
      Windswept deformity (combination of valgus deformity of 1 leg with varus deformity of the other leg)
      Anterior bowing of the tibia and femur
      Coxa vara.
d. Serum calcium—normal or decreased
   Serum phosphorus—decreased (except in CRF)
   Serum alkaline phosphatase—increased.

A 23:

a. Corpus callosum.
b. Lateral ventricle.
c. Third ventricle.

A 24:

a. Right intraventricular opacity
   Right periventricular echogenicity.
b. Right sided grade IV intraventricular hemorrhage.
c. Grade I—Confined to germinal matrix
   Grade II—Intraventricular without ventricular dilatation
   Grade III—Intraventricular with ventricular dilatation
   Grade IV—Periventricular hemorrhagic infarction.

A 25:

a. Bilateral parenchymal cysts.
b. Cystic PVL.
c. Intraventricular hemorrhage/ischemia.

A 26:

a. Right clavicular fracture.
b. Brachial plexus injury.

A 27:

a. Respiratory distress syndrome.
b. Fine reticulogranular opacities
   Air bronchogram.
c. Antenatal steroids.

A 28:

a. Hyperinflated lung fields
   Fluid in horizontal fissure.
b. Transient tachypnea of newborn
c. Good
d. No.

A 29:

a. Bilateral coarse opacities.
b. Meconium aspiration syndrome.
c. Intubation
   Ventilation
   IV Dextrose bolus
   IV Normal saline bolus.

A 30:

a. Pneumopericardium.
b. ECG—low voltage, positive transillumination.
c. Needle aspiration.
d. Conservative management.

A 31:

a. No pulmonary tissue or bronchial markings seen on right side
   Mediastinal shift to the right
   Crowding of ribs on right side.
b. Agenesis of right lung.
c. VACTERL sequence
   Ipsilateral facial and skeletal malformations
   Central nervous system malformations
   Cardiac malformations.

A 32:

a. Eventration of the diaphragm.
b. CT Chest.

A 33:

a. Scoliosis.
b. Idiopathic thoracic curvatures may not create significant alterations in cardiopulmonary function until they have reached 80-90°.
c. Cardiopulmonary compromise
   Difficulty in walking
   (Most common indication is cosmetic deformity).
d. *Congenital,* e.g. Failure of formation—Wedge vertebrae, hemivertebrae
   Neuromuscular Neuropathic diseases
   　　Poliomyelitis
   　　Spinocerebellar degeneration (Friedreich ataxia, Charcot Marie—Tooth disease)
   　　Syringomyelia
   　　Spinal cord tumor
   　　Spinal cord trauma
   　　Spinal muscular atrophy
   　　Duchenne muscular dystrophy
   　　Arthrogryposis.
   Syndromes e.g. Neurofibromatosis, Marfan syndrome.
   Idiopathic.

A 34:

a. Transposition of great arteries.
b. Egg on side appearance.
c. Prostaglandin E_1.
d. Rashkind balloon atrial septostomy.
e. Jantene: Arterial switch procedure—usually within first 2 to 4 weeks of life
   Mustard procedure.

A 35:

a. Tetrology of Fallot.
b. "Coeur en sabot"- boot shaped heart.
c. Ejection systolic murmur heard best in left upper sternal edge.
   Single second heart sound.
d. Cerebral thrombosis
   Brain abscess.

A 36:

a. Supracardiac TAPVD.
b. "Snowman sign".
c. Mild cyanosis
   Cardiac failure
   Recurrent chest infection
   Pulmonary hypertension.

Renal System

QUESTIONS

Q1. Metabolic compensation of respiratory disorders.

Disorder	
Acute respiratory acidosis	(HCO_3^-) increase by___ for each _____ increase in (P_{CO2})
Chronic respiratory acidosis	(HCO_3^-) increase by___ for each _____ increase in (P_{CO2})
Acute respiratory alkalosis	(HCO_3^-) decrease by___ for each _____ decrease in (P_{CO2})
Chronic respiratory alkalosis	(HCO_3^-) decrease by___ for each _____ decrease in (P_{CO2})

Q2. You receive KUB ultrasound report of a 4-year-old child. His height is 100 cm and weight is 22 kg. His serum creatinine is 1.

a. What is his approximate bladder capacity?
b. What is the volume considered to be significant for post void urine?
c. You suspect a renal tract abnormality, what is the investigation of choice to rule out scarring?
d. Calculate his GFR using Schwartz formula.

Q3. Fractional excretion of sodium. Give below is the serum and urinary electrolyte report of a 6-year-old child.

UNa+	100
UCr	90
UCL⁻	90
UK⁺	25
S Na⁺	135
SCr	1
SCL⁻	100
S K⁺	4

a. Calculate FeNa
b. FeNa is_____than 1% with acute tubular necrosis.
c. FeNa is_____than 1% with severe obstruction of the urinary drainage of both kidneys.
d. FeNa is_____than 1% with acute glomerulonephritis.
e. FeNa is_____than 1% with hepatorenal syndrome.
f. FeNa is_____than 1% with states of prerenal azotemia such as congestive heart failure or dehydration.

Q4. Serum osmolality. Attached are serum reports of a 7 year old.

S Na$^+$	140 mEq/L
S Cr	1
SCL$^-$	100 mEq/L
S K$^+$	4 mEq/L
S Glucose	90 mg/dL
BUN	14 mg/dL

a. Calculate his serum osmolality?
b. What is the normal range?

Q5. Serum Na-136, Cl-102 and HCO$_3$-10
a. What is the anion gap?
b. What is the normal anion gap?
c. What is the likely anion gap in following (normal or increased)?
  i. Diarrhea
  ii. Lactic acidosis
  iii. DKA
  iv. ARF
  v. RTA
  vi. Salicylate poisoning
  vii. Urinary tract diversion
  viii. IEM
  ix. Septic shock
  x. Post hypocapnea.

Q6. A 9-month-old male infant is admitted in PICU with bacterial meningitis. His mean BP is 38 mm Hg. His laboratory reports are as follows.

Serum sodium	: 126 meq/L
Serum potassium	: 4.2 meq/L
Urine output	: 4.7 mL/kg/h
Urinary sodium	: 151 meq/L

a. What is the cause of hyponatremia in this child?
b. List 2 investigations which will help in confirming the diagnosis.
c. How will you correct the electrolyte imbalance?
d. List two symptoms of hyponatremia.

Q7. Given below are the reports of a 4-year-old male child admitted with a diagnosis of severe pneumonia. He is neurologically normal and has a urine output of 1.2 mL/kg/hr. His laboratory reports are as follows.

Serum sodium	:	129 meq/L
Serum potassium	:	4.1 meq/L
Urinary sodium	:	31 meq/L
Urinary potassium	:	12 meq/L

a. What is most likely condition causing this electrolyte abnormality?
b. List 4 causes other than pneumonia which can lead into this condition.
c. How will you treat this condition?

Q8. 3-year-old male child presented in pediatric OPD with a history of 1 episode of abnormal movement 2 hours back. Parents also give history of oliguria and irritability for past 36 hours. He also has a 3-day history of bloody stools which stopped 3 days back. Parents were giving ORS for past 3 days. On examination, he is pale, edematous, hepatomegaly, and has petchiae all over the body. His HR is 140/min, BP is 100/60 mm Hg. His arterial blood gas shows mild metabolic acidosis.

a. What is the most likely diagnosis?
b. What is the most likely etiology/pathogen involved in the above diagnosis?
c. List two differential diagnoses.
d. List 2 electrolyte abnormalities which can be associated with this diagnosis.

Q9. Study the DTPA scan shown below and answer the questions.

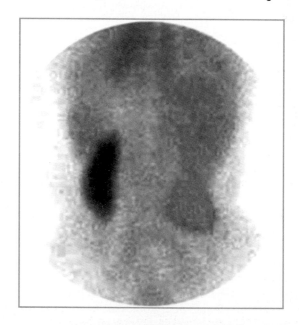

a. What is the diagnosis on this DTPA scan?
b. What do the DTPA and DMSA stand for?

Q10. A 12-year-old boy is brought to the clinic with recurrent cramps. On examination, his growth is normal. He is normotensive and has no evidence of rickets. His systemic examination is normal. His laboratory reports are as follows.

Hb	:	12.1 g/dL
BUN	:	8 mg/dL
Serum creatinine	:	0.4 mg/dL
Serum sodium	:	141 meq/L
Serum potassium	:	2.5 meq/L
Serum chloride	:	90 meq/L
Serum magnesium	:	0.5 mmol/L (low)
Urinary chloride	:	35 meq/L
Blood gas		
pH	:	7.52
HCO_3	:	30 meq/l

a. What is the most probable diagnosis?
b. What is the mode of inheritance?
c. What is the treatment?

Q11. Match the following.

Histology	Glomerular pathology
a. Diffuse mesangial proliferative	1. Alport syndrome
b. Focal segmental	2. IGA nephropathy
c. With crescents	3. RPGN
d. Foam cells	4. Poststreptococcal

Q12. A 16-year-old female, known case of SLE presents to pediatric OPD with intermittent hemoptysis and hematuria. On examination, she is noted to be pale and hypertensive. On investigation, her complement levels were normal. Further investigation revealed antibodies to lung and glomerular basement membrane.

a. What is the most likely diagnosis?
b. What is the most likely cause of hemoptysis in this patient?
c. List 2 treatment options.

Q13. A 3-year-old female child is reviewed in pediatric OPD for failing to thrive and abdominal pain. Her investigation revealed Hb 10 g/dL, serum sodium of 136 meq/L, serum potassium of 2.9 meq/L and metabolic acidosis. Her urinary pH was 6.1. On further evaluation, she is diagnosed to have renal stones.

a. What is the most likely diagnosis including the subtype of the pathology?
b. What is the underlying pathogenesis?
c. What is the treatment?

Q14. A 2-year-old female child is reviewed in pediatric OPD for short stature. She also complains of polyuria and polydipsia. Her examination revealed signs of rickets. Her investigation showed serum sodium of

137 meq/L, serum potassium of 2.8 meq/L and metabolic acidosis. Her urinary pH was 4.9. On further evaluation, she is diagnosed to have renal stones.

a. What is the most likely diagnosis including the subtype of the pathology?
b. What is the underlying pathogenesis?
c. What is the treatment?

Q15. Given below is the photograph of an 8-day-old male neonate. He is also diagnosed to have undescended testis and urinary tract abnormality.

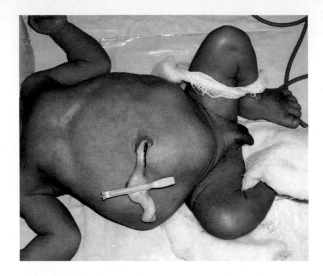

a. What is the diagnosis?
b. What are the associated urinary tract abnormalities with this condition?
c. Give 1 pulmonary complication associated with this condition.

Q16. 4-year-old child with nephrotic syndrome presents with fever, vomiting, severe abdominal pain and abdominal distension. On examination, his HR is 160/min along with shallow and rapid breathing. His blood tests reveal peripheral leucocytosis with a marked predominance of polymorphonuclear cells.

a. What is the diagnosis?
b. How would you confirm the diagnosis?
c. What is the most likely cause/pathogen/organism for the same?
d. What is the immediate treatment?

Q17. A 1½-years-old child presents with failure to thrive muscle weakness, constipation and polyuria. His arterial blood gas shows:

pH   : 7.57
pCO_2 : 36
pO_2 : 78
HCO_3^- : 38
Saturation : 98%

a. What is your interpretation of the ABG?
b. List 4 clinical conditions in which this ABG finding can be seen.
   On further investigation, he was noted to have hypokalemia.
c. List 2 possible diagnoses.
   His urine shows hypercalciuria.
d. What is the diagnosis?
e. How do you treat this patient?

Q18. A 3-year-old female presented to pediatric OPD with complaint of irritability and lethargy. On examination, she appears pale. On further questioning mother gave history of URTI 1 week back for which she consulted a local physician who conservatively treated it as viral URI. She also gave history of decreased urine output. After a week of the above illness, she became irritable and lethargic. Childs blood investigations revealed a BUN of 81 mg/dL and serum creatinine of 4.2 mg/dL. Her blood gas shows pH of 7.18 and serum K of 5.6 mmol/dL with tall T waves in the ECG. Her platelet count is 85,000/mm.

a. What is the diagnosis?
b. What are the possible findings on the peripheral smear of this child?
c. What is the most common organism associated with this disease?
d. List 2 indications of dialysis in this child.

Q19. Given below is the picture of a 6-year-old boy presenting in OPD with complaint of severe abdominal pain of 1 day duration. On examination, he is noted to have similar rash over buttocks and thighs. His CBC and clotting profile is normal.

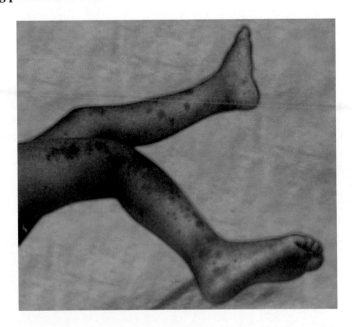

a. What is the most likely diagnosis?
b. What is the prognosis?
c. What are the factors associated with worst prognosis?
d. List 2 possible long-term complications.

Q20. What is the dietary requirement for a child with acute renal failure in terms of:

a. Calorie requirement.
b. Protein requirement.
c. Sodium requirement.
d. Potassium intake.
e. Phosphorus.

ANSWERS

A 1:

Disorder	
Acute respiratory acidosis	(HCO_3^-) increase by 1 for each 10 mm Hg increase in (PCO_2)
Chronic respiratory acidosis	(HCO_3^-) increase by 3.5 for each 10 mm Hg increase in (PCO_2) 4
Acute respiratory alkalosis	(HCO_3^-) decrease by 2 for each 10 mm Hg decrease in (PCO_2) 1-3
Chronic respiratory alkalosis	(HCO_3^-) decrease by 4 for each 10 mm Hg decrease in (PCO_2) 2-5

A 2:

a. (Age + 2) × 30
    180 mL
b. 44 mL (25 mL or 2 mL/kg) ????   How 25 mL??
c. DMSA
d. 0.55 × Ht (cm)
    Serum Creatinine
    $$\frac{0.55 \times 100}{1}$$
    55 mL/min per 1.73 m².

A 3:

a. 0.8%

$$FeNa = \frac{U_{Na} * P_{Cr}}{P_{Na} * U_{Cr}} \times 100$$

b. Greater
c. Greater
d. Less
e. Less
f. Less.

A 4:

a. 285.5

$$Osmolality = 2 * Na + \frac{Glu}{18} + \frac{BUN}{2.8}$$

b. 275–290.

A 5:

a. $(136) - (102 + 10) = 24$
b. 8–16
c.

     i.   Diarrhea—normal
     ii. Lactic acidosis—increased
     iii. DKA—increased
     iv. ARF—increased
     v.   RTA—normal
     vi. Salicylate—increased
     vii. Urinary tract diversion—normal
    viii. IEM—increased
     ix. Septic shock—increased
     x.   Post hypocapnea—normal.

A 6:

a. Cerebral salt wasting.
b. Serum uric acid, serum vasopressin level.
c. 3% NaCl.
    Treatment of patients with cerebral salt wasting consists of restoring intravascular volume with sodium chloride and water, as for the treatment of other causes of systemic dehydration. The underlying cause of the disorder, which is usually due to acute brain injury, should also be treated if possible. Treatment involves the ongoing replacement of urine sodium losses (volume for volume).
d. Convulsion, irritability, alteration of sensorium.

A 7:

a. SIADH.
b. 1. Excessive administration of vasopressin in the treatment of central diabetes insipidus
    2. Encephalitis
    3. Brain tumors
    4. Head trauma
    5. Psychiatric disease
    6. Postictal period after generalized seizures
    7. After prolonged nausea
    8. Tuberculous meningitis, and with
    9. AIDS
    10. Hypothalamic-pituitary surgery
    11. Drugs—oxcarbazepine, carbamazepine, chlorpropamide, vinblastine, vincristine, and tricyclic antidepressants.
c. Fluid restriction
    SIADH is characterized by hyponatremia, an inappropriately concentrated urine (>100 mOsm/kg), normal or slightly elevated plasma volume, normal-to-high urine sodium, and low serum uric acid.

A 8:

a. Hemolytic uremic syndrome.
b. *E. coli*—0157: H7.
c. 1. Acute glomerulonephritis
   2. Dyselectrolytemia
   3. Intussusception.
d. Hyponatremia/hypernatremia/hyperkalemia.

A 9:

a. Absent left sided kidney perfusion.
b. DTPA   : ^{99}Tc labeled diethylenetriaminepentaacetic
   acid scan
   DMSA   :   Dimercaptosuccinic acid scan

A 10:

a. Gitelman's syndrome.
b. Autosomal recessive.
c. Potassium and magnesium supplements.

A 11:

Histology	Glomerular pathology
a. Diffuse mesangial proliferative	Post streptococcal
b. Focal segmental	IGA nephropathy
c. With crescents RPGN	RPGN
d. Foam cells	Alport syndrome

A 12:

a. Goodpasture disease.
b. Pulmonary hemorrhage.
c. Pulsed methylprednisolone
   Immunosuppression-cyclophosphamide
   Plasmapheresis.

A 13:

a. Type I or distal RTA.
b. Impaired distal urinary acidification/H$^+$ion secretion.
c. Bicarbonate supplementation, thiazide diuretics.

A 14:

a. Type II or proximal RTA.
b. Impaired distal urinary acidification/H$^+$ion secretion.
c. Bicarbonate supplementation.

A 15:

a. Prune-Belly syndrome (Eagle-Barrett syndrome).
b. Dilated ureter (megaureter), megalourethra
   Large bladder.
c. Pulmonary hypoplasia.

A 16:

a. Spontaneous bacterial peritonitis.
b. Ascitic tap-PMN >250 cells/μL, with PMNs ≥ 50%, is presumptive evidence of SBP.
c. Pneumococci.
d. Parenteral antibiotic therapy with cefotaxime and an aminoglycoside.

A 17:

a. Metabolic alkalosis uncompensated.
b. Gastric losses (emesis or nasogastric suction)
   Diuretics
   Gitelman syndrome
   Bartter syndrome
   Base administration
   Autosomal dominant hypoparathyroidism
   Adrenal adenoma or hyperplasia
   Glucocorticoid-remedial aldosteronism
   Renovascular disease
   Renin-secreting tumor
   Cushing syndrome
c. Gitelman syndrome
   Bartter syndrome.
d. Bartter syndrome.
e. Potassium supplementation, adequate hydration, nutritional supplementation. Indomethacin might be used.

A 18:

a. Hemolytic-uremic syndrome atypical presentation: More commonly presents following gastroenteritis but occasionally can be following URI.
b. Peripheral smear: Burr cell, helmet cell, fragmented RBCs, leucocytosis, thrombocytopenia.
c. *E. coli* 0157: H7 (~70–80% of HUS).
d. Seizures
   pH <7.2
   K 5.5–6.0 with ECG changes.

A 19:

a. Henöch-Schonlein purpura.
b. Generally favorable 97–98%.
c. Acute nephritic and/or nephrotic syndrome.
d. Hypertension
   Pregnancy-induced hypertension
   Hematuria
   Chronic renal failure.

A 20:

a. Calories-maximized—at least the daily requirement of 100 kcal/kg/day.
b. Protein—restrict moderately.
c. Sodium—restrict, restrict salt—no added salt.
d. Potassium—restrict, avoid K containing food.
e. Phosphorus—restrict.

Orthopedics

QUESTIONS

Q1.

a. What major problems can occur in using a cast?
b. What are the signs that the cast is too tight?
c. How do you prevent a tight cast?
d. How long does it take for a cast to harden?

Q2.

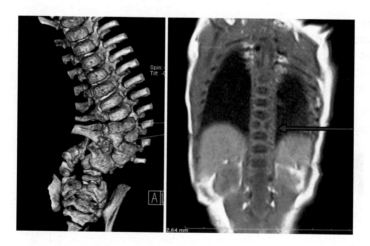

a. What is the radiological anomaly?
b. What is the incidence?
    i. 1:300
    ii. 1:3000
    iii. 1:30000
    iv. 1:300000
c. What can be the clinical abnormality associated with above abnormality?

Q3.

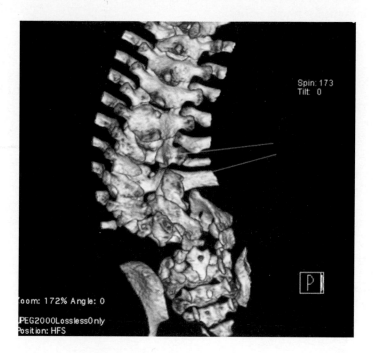

a. What is the radiological finding?
b. What is the diagnosis?
c. What are common physical signs of above diagnosis?
d. What is the single most important prenatal/antenatal factor leading into above abnormality?

Q4. A 10-year-old presents with history of weakness in the legs; low back pain; scoliosis; and incontinence.

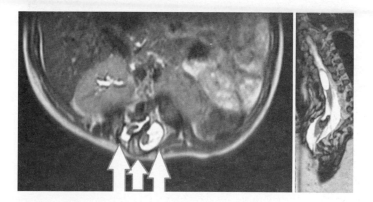

a. What is the radiological finding?
b. What is the diagnosis?
c. What is the treatment?

Q5. Attached are pre and 2 weeks postoperative X-rays of a baby with development dysplasia of hip.

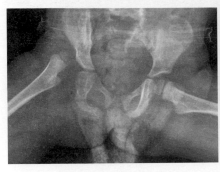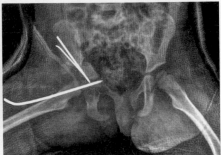

a. Which of the following is a risk factor for DDH? True/False
   i. First born
   ii. Male
   iii. Family history of DDH
   iv. Breech.
b. Enlist 2 orthopedic conditions associated with DDH
c. Name 2 screening tests on examinations used to confirm the diagnosis.

Q6.

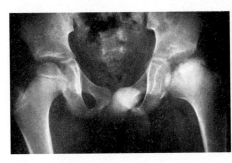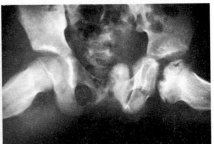

a. What are the radiological findings?
b. What is the diagnosis?
c. What is the pathological process?
d. True false
   i. Most commonly occur in children of 5–9 years age.
   ii. Is more common in females?
   iii. Is more common in children who have a sedentary lifestyle?
   iv. Surgical correction is most common modality of treatment.

Q7. Attached are MRI images of an 8-year-old female.

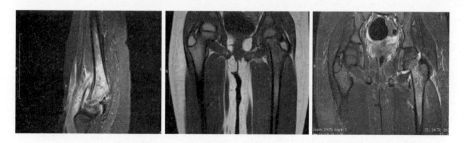

a. What are the radiological findings?
b. What is the diagnosis?
c. What is the treatment?
d. Enlist 3 complications associated with above diagnosis.

Q8.

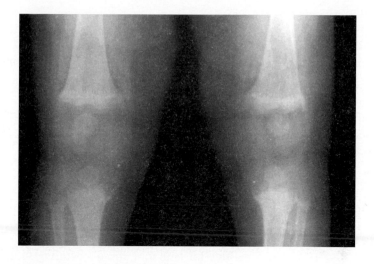

a. What is the diagnosis?
b. This infant is 10 months old, what is the most likely sub type?
c. What is the earliest sign of this disorder?
d. What is the first radiological change that occurs in response to specific therapy?
e. How could this have been prevented?
f. What are the non-specific urinary findings in this disorder? (at least 2).

ANSWERS

A 1:

a. A cast that is too tight can cause serious neurovascular compromise.

b.
  - Pain when moving the figures/toes
  - Pallor, or pale/white distal part due to lack of blood supply
  - Paresthesias and possible numbness due to nerve compression and lack of circulation
  - Paralysis due to loss of nerve function.

c.
  - Use sufficient padding
  - Split the cast on both sides and spread the cast to allow for swelling (bivalving)
  - Split the padding to the skin
  - Elevate the limb to prevent dependent edema and inflammatory swelling

d. Plaster cast   2–8 minutes
   Fiber glass   4–5 minutes

A 2:

a. Hemi vertebrae-fusion defect of marked vertebrae
b. B (1:3000)
c. Kyphosis- DORSAL
   Scoliosis
   Lordosis

A 3:

a. Unfused posterior element of marked vertebrae
b. Spina bifida
c.
  i. Leg weakness and paralysis
  ii. Orthopedic abnormalities, i.e. club foot, hip dislocation, scoliosis
  iii. Bladder and bowel control problems, including incontinence, urinary tract infections, and poor kidney function
  iv. Pressure sores and skin irritations
  v. Abnormal eye movement
c. Not having enough folic acid during pregnancy.

A 4:

a. Bony spur noted between 2 divided cords
b. Diastematomyelia
c. Surgery-decompression (surgery) of neural elements and removal of bony spur.

A 5:

a.
   i. True
   ii. False
   iii. True
   iv. True.
b. Torticollis, congenital hyperextension of knee, club foot, skull and facial deformities.
c. Ortolani
   Barlows

Note: Please practise ortolani and Barlows manuver as these can be asked for demonstration in observed OSCE stations.

A 6:

a. Uniformly increased density of left femoral head.
b. Legg-calve-perthes disease.
c. Idiopathic avascular necrosis of femoral head.
d.
   i. True
   ii. False
   iii. False
   iv. False.

A 7:

a. Heterogenous hyperintense signal of neck and upper end of femur.
b. Osteomyelitis.
c. Antimicrobial therapy.
d.
   • Septic arthritis
   • Distant seeding leading into pneumonia, septic pericarditis, etc.
   • Pathological fracture
   • Physeal bars
   • Recurrent infections.

A 8:

a. Rickets
b. Vitamin D deficiency
c. Craniotabes
d. Appearance of provisional zone of classification
e. Supplement of 400IU of vitamin D from birth
f. Generalized aminoaciduria
   • Glycosuria
   • Phosphaturia
   • Elevated urinary citrate
   • Impaired renal acidification.

Device and Equipments

QUESTIONS

Q1.

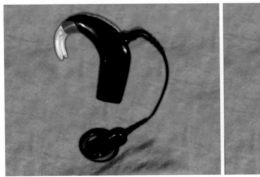

a. Name the device seen in the picture.
b. What are the essential parts of the device?
c. Enlist 3 commonest types of devices available.

Q2.

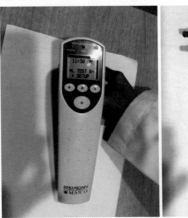
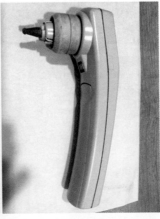

a. Name the device seen in the picture.
b. Which organ function does it detect?
c. How does this device work?
d. What are the prerequisite and limitations of working of the device?

Q3.

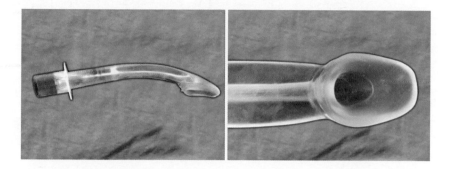

a. Name the device
b. Indication
c. Complication
d. Contraindication when above device shall be avoided in a child during elective procedure.

Q4. Check functionality of self inflating bag.

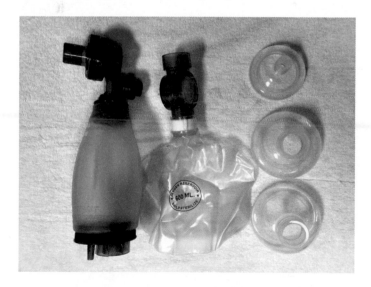

Q5.

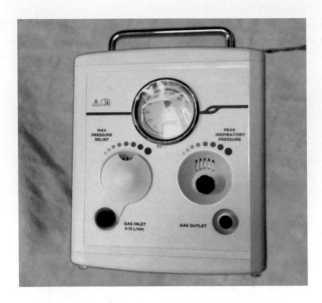

    i. Name the device
   ii. Name the controls
  iii. What is the advantage and disadvantage over self inflating bag.

Q6.

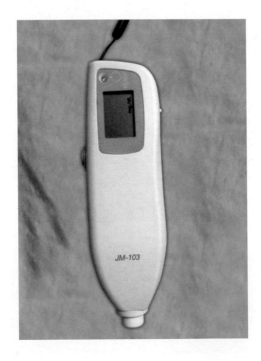

a. What is the device shown?
b. What is the site of use?
c. What are the single most important advantage and limitation of use?

Q7. Name the device shown?

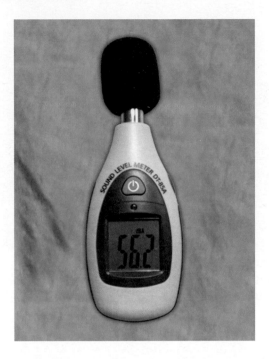

Q8. Name the device shown?

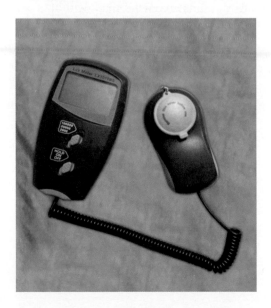

Q9.

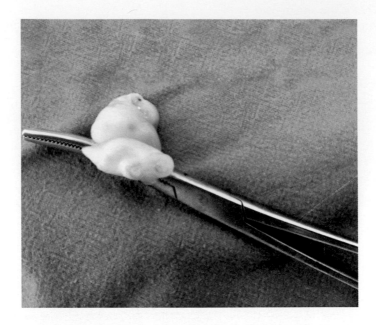

a. What is the abnormality seen?
b. What is the incidence?
    i. 1:10
    ii. 1:100
    iii. 1:1000
    iv. 1:10000
    v. 1:100000.
c. It is associated with other anomalies in.
    i. 1% cases
    ii. 10% cases
    iii. 25% cases
    iv. 50% cases
    v. 75% cases
d. What are the 2 most common systems involved in associated anomalies?

Q10.

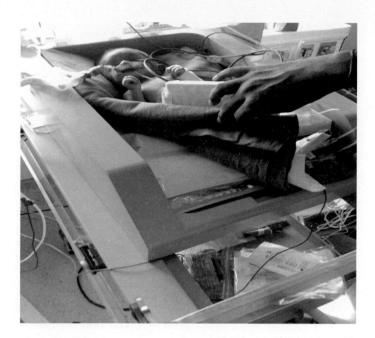

a. What procedure is this baby undergoing?
b. Name the device.
c. Enlist 5 complications associated with above procedure.

Q11. A lumbar puncture is performed.

a. The CSF is xanthochromatic. What are the four possible causes?
b. CSF protein levels are 350 mg/dL. What are the three possible causes for the same?
c. CSF glucose in 210 mg/dL and blood glucose is 118 mg/dL. List five causes for the same.
d. CSF is cloudy, what is the likely cause?

ANSWERS

A 1:

a. Hearing aid

b.
- Microphone
- Amplifier
- Receiver
- Microchip
- Battery.

c.
- Invisible
- Behind the ear
- In the ear canal.

A 2:

a. Oto acoustic emission (OAE) testing device.

b. Inner ear.

c. In healthy cochlea, vibration of the hair cells in response to noise generates the acoustic energy-called oto acoustic emission. Probe is placed in ear canal and generates a click. The energy produced is detected by a microphone within the probe.

d. Needs quite baby.

No debris in ear canal; chances of false positivity high if performed in first 24 hours of birth due to chances of presence of vernix or other debris in the ear canal.

Only assess function of ear- no assessment of neural pathway.

Its a screening test. Failed OAE should be confirmed by BERA later.

A 3:

a. Laryngeal mask airway

b. Indication
- Difficult airway
- Routine airway opening
- Pre hospital airway management.

c. Complication
- Aspiration
- Dislodgement
- Upper airway trauma.

c. Contraindication
- Complete upper airway obstruction
- Increased risk of aspiration
    - Prolonged bag-valve-mask ventilation
    - Patients who have not fasted before ventilation
    - Upper gastrointestinal bleed.
- Suspected or known abnormalities in supraglottic anatomy
- Need for high airway pressures.

A 4:

- Assemble the device correctly.
- With a flow/self inflating bag occlude the face mask against the palm.
- Look for following of features as you squeeze the bag—
    a. You should feel pressure against the palm.
    b. The fish mouth valve should open and close.
    c. The pop off valve should make a hissing sound or move up and down.
    d. The bag should recoil instantly when pressure is released.
    e. If a pressure manometer is attached it should display the pressure when bag is squeezed.
    Absence of any of the above feature suggests malfunction.

A 5:

i. *T-piece resuscitator x`*
ii.
- The inspiratory pressure control—sets the amount of pressure delivered during a normal assisted breath.
- The maximum pressure relief control is a safety feature that prevents the pressure from exceeding a preset value (usually 40 cm H_2O, but adjustable).

iii.

Advantages

1. Consistent delivery of PIP and PEEP.
2. Can be used to provide free flow oxygen reliably—21–100 % (with blender)
3. Provider does not get tired from ventilation.

Disadvantages

1. Needs compressed gas with a blender.
2. Requires pressures to be set prior to use.
3. Changing inflation pressure during resuscitation is more difficult.
4. Risks of prolonged inspiratory time.

A 6:

a. Transcutaneous bilirubinometer.
b. Forehead and the upper end of sternum.
c. Non invasive.
   Cannot be used in babies' already receiving/received phototherapy (unless the area is covered during treatment).

A 7:

Sound level monitor.

A 8:

Flux meter.

A 9:

a. Single umbilical artery
b. B
c. C
d. Genitourinary followed by cardiovascular and musculoskeletal.

A 10:

a. Therapeutic hypothermia.
b. Whole body cooling device.
c.

- Delayed intracardiac conduction with sinus bradycardia
- Prolonged QT interval
- Ventricular arrhythmias
- Reduced cardiac output
- Hypotension
- Reduction in surfactant production
- Increase pulmonary vascular resistance
- Increase oxygen consumption and oxygen requirement
- Affects coagulation cascade and viscosity—coagulopathy that may be complicated by thrombus or hemorrhage
- Anemia
- Thrombocytopenia
- Leukopenia–increase risk of sepsis
- Renal impairment
- Metabolic and lactic acidosis
- Hypokalemia
- Hypoglycemia
- Impaired liver function.

A 11:

a.

- Hyperbilirubinemia
- Subarachnoid hemorrhage
- Markedly elevated CSF protein
- Carotenemia.

b.

- TB meningitis
- GBS
- Tumors of spinal cord or brain
- Degenerative disorders
- Vasculitis
- Multiple sclerosis.

c.

- Bacterial meningitis
- TBM
- Fungal meningitis
- Aseptic meningitis
- Neoplasms of meninges.

d. Elevated cell count—WBC or RBC
- Name the device
- Enlist 5 common complications associated with the device
- Name the commonest hazard associated with malfunctioning of device and remediate actions
- Enlist 5 indications of usage.

Chapter
22

Ophthalmology/Eye

QUESTIONS

Q1.

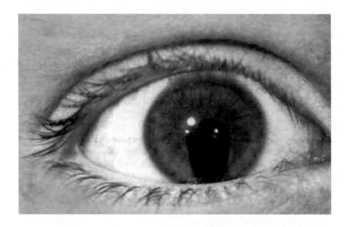

a. What is the diagnosis?
b. Enlist 2 acquired and 2 congenital conditions leading into this eye problem.
c. What can be the clinical symptoms due to above defect?

Q2.

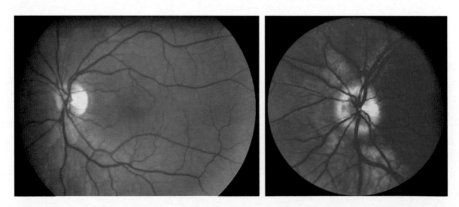

a. Describe the eye findings.
b. Enlist three cause.

Q3. A 2-month-old infant presents with bilateral cataracts.

a. What is the most common indentifiable inheritance pattern for bilateral cataracts?
b. Enlist 2 other common causes of bilateral cataracts.
c. What is the optimum time to operate on a patient with bilateral dense congenital cataracts?
d. What is the preferred treatment for congenital cataracts in a 2-month-old infant with compliant parents?
e. What can be the complications if it is left untreated?

Q4. Select the answers

a. Kayser-Fleisher rings
b. Cherry red macular spots
c. Kinky hair
d. Arcus juvenilis
   i. Familial hypercholesterolemia
   ii. Tay-Sachs diseased
   iii. Wilson diseases
   iv. Menkes syndrome.

ANSWERS

A 1:

a. Coloboma (iris) of right eye
b. Acquired
    - Eye surgery
    - Trauma to the eye.

    Congenital
    - CHARGE syndrome
    - Cat eye syndrome
    - Patau syndrome
    - Treacher Collins syndrome.
c. Blurred vision
    Decreased visual acuity
    Double vision
    Ghost image.

A 2:

a. Papilloedemea   Erythema
                        Swelling of disc
                        Blaring of margins
b. Optic atrophy   Pale discs

A 3:

a. Autosomal dominant
b. Diabetes mellitus, galactosemia, Lowe's syndrome
c. As soon as possible
d. Lensectomy, anterior vitrectomy, and fitting of contact lens
e. Irreversible ambylopia and sensory nystagmus.

A 4:

a. 3
b. 2
c. 4
d. 1.